AFRICAN DANCE EDUCATION IN GHANA

AFRICAN DANCE EDUCATION IN GHANA

Curriculum and Instructional Materials for A Model Bachelor of Arts (Hons.) Dance in Society

W. OFOTSU ADINKU

Senior Lecturer, Department of Theatre Arts,
School of Performing Arts, University of Ghana,
Legon, Ghana

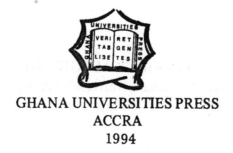

GHANA UNIVERSITIES PRESS
ACCRA
1994

Published by
Ghana Universities Press
P. O. Box GP 4219
Accra.

Tel. 233 (21) 513383, 513401/4
Fax 233 (021) 513402

First published in 1994, Reprinted 2009
© W. Ofotsu Adinku, 1994
ISBN: 9964–3–0205–3

PRODUCED IN GHANA
Typeset by Ghana Universities Press, Accra
Printed by Assemblies of God Literature Centre, Limited, Accra.

CONTENTS

PREFACE

For a dance to be developed to acquire a Ghanaian and an African character, dance developers will need to draw on models of our total cultural inheritance. Until the wellsprings of the dance cultures are made to nourish our new dance forms, we cannot describe our developments as healthy.

In the light of the above, dance educators, planners, performers and choreographers who set their minds on new developments of dances for the emergent theatre and education system must reshape the old model into new forms. The dance developers need education in the essences of the traditional dances as well as in creative issues to enable them to meet the challenges of our new cultural and educational evolution. In this book, therefore, suggestions have been made to enhance the old teaching system that operates at the diploma level, and a sample of a curriculum has been drawn up to meet the training and educational needs of our dance developers.

It is hoped that the book will be read by teachers of dance, students, dance researchers and those whose responsibilities are in preparing a curriculum for academic awards in African dance. Others such as practitioners of dance as a non-examinable subject will profit by reading the book.

I am grateful to all those whose ideas and works have influenced my thinking. In particular, I express my gratitude and appreciation to Professor June Layson and Dr. Janet Adshead (both of the University of Surrey, United Kingdom) whose encouragement, guidance and contributions resulted in the writing of a Ph.D thesis which has now been revised for this book. Professor Layson and Dr. Adshead showed a good deal of motherly interest and love in my studies and were always ready to offer their precious hours in advising and counselling me.

I wish to acknowledge the tremendous assistance given me by David Henshaw, former Principal Lecturer, and Head of Dance Department, Middlesex Polytechnic, London. He was my source of inspiration and financial support, and allowed me to live in his

vii

London flat whenever I needed it. I wish him Peace Profound.

I acknowledge with gratitude financial support from the University of Ghana for studentship at the University of Surrey, Guildford, United Kingdom from 1983 to 1986 to pursue a research interest.

My greatest debt is to Professor J. H. Kwabena Nketia, former Director of the Institute of African Studies and the School of Music, Dance and Drama, and Professor Albert Mawere Opoku, former Head of Dance and Artistic Director of the National Dance Company (Ghana Dance Ensemble), University of Ghana, for introducing me to the values of African dance in education and theatre practice.

School of Performing Arts   W. OFOTSU ADINKU
University of Ghana
Legon
10th January, 1990

INTRODUCTION

In fulfilment of the desire to introduce traditional aesthetic forms into new creative developments in Ghana, the Government came out with the concept of the National Theatre Movement (Hammond, 1977, p.7). The concept was based on the notion that school-educated personalities, who were the symbols of change in the new artistic community envisaged for the country, should become aware of traditional aesthetic forms. They should, therefore, employ models of these traditional forms for new developments to meet the growing aspirations of the people; otherwise, the country would be bound to rely on foreign artistic forms, some of which, in the long run, would be detrimental to the progress of artistic-conscious Ghanaians. In order to forstall this problem, the implementation of the objectives of the concept of National Theatre Movement was deemed appropriate. Accordingly, traditional creative activities became part of classroom learning.

The term 'creative culture' has a definition which, according to Nketia (1976, p.3), includes literature, visual arts and performing arts. Literature in the traditional society operates in oral forms such as story-telling, proverbs and wise sayings; visual arts include painting, sculpture and pottery, while the performing arts embrace mostly dance, music, and drama.

The study and development of various aspects of the creative culture was assigned to the Institute of African Studies at the University of Ghana in October, 1962. Within the Institute of African Studies was the School of Music and Drama[1] whose Research Fellows were charged by Government with the responsibility of carrying out research and offering instruction in the traditional performing arts, as well as establishing processess for the development of new arts forms based on traditional models. Dance development and education played a significant role in the School of Music and Drama under the supervision of Professor J. H. Nketia and Professor A. M. Opoku.

Prior to the establishment of curricula for dance study at

1

the Certificate and Diploma levels at the University of Ghana, Nketia and Opoku, acting on Government policy, helped to establish the National Dance Company.[2] It was these developments and arrangements which ushered in dance as an important aspect of artistic development both in practical and academic activities in the history of cultural development in Ghana.

The writer, by virtue of his pioneering role as a member of the National Dance Company and student of dance and related art forms, discusses in this book some of the programmes offered for the training and education of the dance artist and scholar at the Certificate and Diploma levels. He makes suggestions for the development of a curriculum for the Bachelor of Arts (Hons.) Dance in Society in order to improve upon instruction and practice of African Dance at the University of Ghana.

At the moment, instruction in dance as an academic activity at the University of Ghana is restricted to the Diploma level to serve the interests of students with lesser admission qualifications who need a professional training programme in dance to qualify them for vocational areas in performance and composition. The programme for the first degree being envisaged would cater for students with higher admission qualifications who seek an understanding of dance issues at a level beyond the Diploma. Such a programme would also train students for vocational routes in performance, composition, criticism and movement notation.

Students of other departments of the University of Ghana who need an understanding of African dance issues without necessarily considering vocational routes would benefit from the new degree programme. Hitherto such a programme with concentration in African dance areas did not exist for first degree students because the dance programme was restricted to the diploma level. In addition, to enable students to continue their education in the African dance area at the graduate level, a first degree programme would be a pre-requisite qualification for admission to research studies.

The development of the Bachelor of Arts (Hons.) Dance in Society with concentration on African dance being suggested in this book is based on the aims of the National Theatre Movement which state that new developments in artistic forms must be

2

linked to the forms of the African traditional society. Understanding traditional dance forms is, therefore, a pre-requisite for implementing dance education policy in this country. It is in this light that the pioneering research activities of Nketia and Opoku, the founding fathers of dance education and dance theatre, have become important in influencing further growth in dance.

In their work on African dance in Ghana, Nketia and Opoku have operated within the tenets of the National Theatre Movement. In the estimation of the writer, Nketia and Opoku have done more work on African dance as an art form and as cultural expression generally than anybody else on the African continent.

In terms of research and writing, a greater amount of literature on African dance as cultural material is credited to Nketia. His writings which expose ethnological ideas of traditional dances play important roles in bringing out underlying meanings and methods of the performances. Such underlying meanings of traditional dances in Nketia's writing would be used in part to develop the concept of dance as cultural activity. This concept is discussed in Section 1 of Chapter 2.

In terms of practical activity, the choreographic developments of Opoku is significant for dance education. His application of traditional artistic features into new choreographic art would guide students and choreographers seeking methods for applying traditional models in new choreographic developments. Opoku's approach would be spelt out within the concept of dance as art in Section 2 of Chapter 2.

Appraising and judgement of a dance are a recognized feature of a traditional performance. Since dance education and development in Ghana aim at providing a continuity of traditional dance ideas in addition to examining models of appreciation, the educational programme being sought for African dance at the degree level would be structured on that line. The appreciative aspects, influenced by the research results of Opoku and Nketia, are grouped under the concept of dance as aesthetic activity and discussed in Section 3 of Chapter 2.

The central aim of this book is to examine these three concepts as the potential basis of dance education and curriculum development for African dance studies.

3

The book is divided into five chapters. Each chapter deals with a specific problem. Chapter 1 looks at new development in dance in Ghana with an emphasis on theatrical performance and early dance education. Chapter 2 examines a conceptual framework for the study of traditional dance within the concept of dance as cultural activity. The place of theatrical dance as a genre based on Opoku's development is treated under dance as art, while aesthetic analysis of dance in regard to the understanding of the primary movement material is examined in dance as aesthetic activity. Chapter 3 looks at how characteristics of African dance influence subject developments for dance study at the degree level. Finally, Chapter 4 lays stress on tabulation of subjects developed in Chapter 3 into a curriculum for a three-year programme for the Bachelor of Arts (Hons.) Dance in Society.[3] A possible course outline is also spelt out in the Chapter 4. The concluding chapter, Chapter 5, spells out the writer's proposal for dance education in the University of Ghana and its significance for encouraging academic and creative activities. The writer makes suggestions for maintaining Opoku's experiment and encourages its use for establishing a theatrical genre that is exclusively Ghanaian and African.

The writer intends that this proposal would serve the need of Ghanaian and other African University teachers by offering suggestions for the improvement of the quality of instruction in preparing students to become expert choreographers, performers, dance critics, movement notators, and dance historians.

NOTES

1. The School of Music and Drama has since October, 1977 been known as the School of Performing Arts, and operates separately from the Institute of African Studies.

2. The National Dance Company has been known as the Ghana Dance Ensemble since June, 1965.

3. A similar title is used at the University of Surrey, Guilford, United Kingdom.

Chapter 1

THE DEVELOPMENT OF DANCE EDUCATION

In line with the idea to develop a dance-education programme in Ghana to fulfil the concept of the National Theatre Movement was the establishment of a National Dance Company to serve as a repertory troupe experimenting with traditional dances and their models in new development. The beginning of dance education in the country was linked to the formation of the Company. This chapter examines the development of dance education and its link with the National Dance Company which has been known since June, 1965 as the Ghana Dance Ensemble.

Between June and October, 1962 a series of advertisement appeared in the Ghanaian daily papers inviting applications from young men and women between the ages of eighteen and twenty-five for studentship in dance and theatre studies leading to recruitment into the National Dance Company upon successful completion of a 2-year course. Table 1 shows a copy of the advertisement from the *Daily Graphic* of October 22, 1962.

Since the National Dance Company was not in existence prior to the advertisement and selection of students, it happened that selected candidates formed the nucleus of the Company while at the same time undergoing training.

During the audition which comprised improvising movements to traditional music, tests in traditional dancing, singing and physical tests, thirteen youngmen and women were selected in October, 1962. The women were Matilda Attiane,[1] Patience Abena Kwakwa, Hilda Sowa,[1] Helen Mensah, Edna Mensah, Beatrice Addo, Emmerentia Tamakloe and Lily Acquah-Harrison. The men included Victor Clottey, Thomas Ekow Adi,[1] William Ofotsu Adinku, Frank Kwesi Mensah and Emmanuel Ampofo Duodu. Other members were to be added later and in February, 1963, Godfrey Odokwei Sackeyfio joined the Company.

The idea of the establishment of the Company, according to Opoku (1964, p.15), came from the first President, Dr. Kwame

TABLE 1

*Advertisement Inviting Applications for Studentship in Dance
and Theatre Studies*

INSTITUTE OF ART AND CULTURE
SCHOOL OF MUSIC AND DRAMA

Applications are invited for full-time studentiship in DANCE at £G180 (beginners) and £G240 (intermediate) a year, in the Dance Division of the Ghana School of Music and Drama.

Candidates must have good basic education and aptitude for the dance. They must be not less than 18 years of age or more than 25 years old, and must be prepared to undergo rigorous training for a period of TWO years in dance techniques and theatre studies.

Successful candidates will be expected to join the National Dance Company on completion of their course.

Applications should reach the Secretary, Ghana School of Music and Drama, P. O. Box 19, LEGON, not later than 22nd October.

Nkrumah, and it was in line with his concept of the cultural emancipation of Ghana and Africa. Nkrumah believed that future developments for Ghana should be linked with traditional achievements; that traditional achievements should be thoroughly examined, interpreted and recreated for modern use. Dance fell within this category and Professor J. H. Nketia and Professor A. M. Opoku were asked by Government to find the best ways of using the traditional dances for new artistic development. Consequently, the National Dance Company and the Dance Section were established for research and study into various aspects of Ghanaian and other African dance forms: movement activities, choreographic elements, costume, make-ups, and other dramatic expression, for the theatre and for teaching in schools.

From October, 1962 to October, 1964, members were trained in the techniques of Ghanaian and other African dances, drumming and singing. A selection of dances were made from all the various regions of Ghana and some African countries in order for the trainees to become acquanted with the different and varied movement styles of the dances. Various dance and musical

6

groups were invited to the Institute of African Studies, home of National Dance Company, and taught their arts.

Training was not restricted to the campus of the University of Ghana alone. Trainees were sent to a number of towns and villages to learn the dancing and musical arts in their traditional settings. This was intended to give them a first-hand idea about the connections of the artistic expression to the people's festivals, rituals, puberty rites, hunters' celebrations and funeral ceremonies.

By October, 1964, arrangements for the development of dance as an academic programme in the School of Music and Drama,[2] a division of the Institute of African Studies, had been completed by Nketia and Opoku and a curriculum for a Certificate in Dance came into existence.

At this time, eight of the members of the National Dance Company who had undergone intensive practical training for two years were selected for studentship on a non-residential basis, but continued to maintain their relationship with the Company. Theory classes were held in the School from 8.30 a.m. to 12.30 p.m. while practical training with other members of the Company was reserved for the afternoon session from 2.00 p.m. to 5.30 p.m. Describing the training and academic programme in dance at the University, Opoku, then Artistic Director of the Company and head of the Dance Section said:

> The Dance Section of the School of Music and Drama, Institute of African Studies ... has a programme for the Study of Dance. It has as its first objective, the task of supplying the training that the students need to become disciplined dancers, and teachers of dance.
>
> (Opoku, 1964, p.52)

From October, 1964 to June, 1965, students for the subject were intensely tutored in various areas of dance and related courses. Courses for the final examination for the Certificate in Dance are presented in Table 2.

At the final examination held in the courses stated in Table 2, six out of eight students were successful. The successful ones were Emmanuel Ampofo Duodu, Victor Clottey, Godfrey Odokwei Sackeyfio, William Ofotsu Adinku, Helen Mensah and Lily Acquah-Harrison. Two other students, Patience Abena Kwakwa

7

and Emmerentia Tamakloe, had earlier on in September, 1964 won an American Undergraduate Scholarship for a Bachelor of Arts Degree in Julliard School of Music, but later transferred to the University of California, Los Angeles, and so were not available for the Certificate in Dance courses in Ghana. All the four male students were admitted in October, 1965 to continue studies for the Diploma in Dance which then became residential at the University of Ghana. The two successful young women, Helen Mensah and Lily Acquah-Harrison, withdrew their studentship.

TABLE 2

Courses in the Final Examination for the Certificate in Dance

Written Papers
  (1)   Introduction to Movement Analysis and Notation.
  (2)   Studies in African Dance Forms.
  (3)   Theory of Music.

Practical Examination
  (1)   Exercises and Reading in Labanotation Texts.
  (2)   Studies in African Dance Forms.
  (3)   Composition of Dance based on Studies in African Movements.

Source: University of Ghana, *Regulation and Syllabuses*, 1969, p.11.

Various subject areas were included in the Diploma course, programme and additional instructors and lecturers were brought in to augment the existing faculty. The following were lecturers and instructors and the course then taught are given in brackets; Professor J. H. Nketia (African Dance Forms, Drama in African Societies, Ghanaian Folklore, Traiditional African Songs); Professor A. M. Opoku (Labanotation, African Dance Forms, Movement Aspects of Customary Behaviour; Choreography); Grace Nuamah (Akan Dance and Songs); Seth Kobla Ladzekpo (Ewe Dance and Songs). Instructors and lecturers who joined the School later were: Deborah Bertonoff from Israel (Movement/Dance Technique); Drid-Williams from USA (Principles of Choreo-

8

graphy, Dance History and Criticism, Modern Dance Technique);
Odette Blum from USA (Labanotation, Modern Dance Technique);
Professor N. Z. Nayo (Theory of Music) and Sophia D. Lokko
(Dance and the Theatre). Those who taught on part-time basis
included B. S. Kwakwa (English Language) and Ama Aidoo
(English Language).

Various drummers and musicians were also engaged on the
basis of their areas of specialization. Their main jobs were in the
Company but they also instructed students in drumming and
singing. Among them were Iddrisu Alhassan (Dagbani Music);
J. Asmah (Ahanta Music); John Bennisan[3] (Togo-Ewe Music);
Seth Kobla Ladzekpo (Anlo-Ewe Music); Husunu Afadi (Anlo-Ewe
Music); Mustapha Tettey Addy (Ga-Dangme Music); Osei Bonsu
(Ashanti Music) and Kwesi Badu (Ashanti Music).

The admittance into full-time courses of some of the
members did not make them sever their link with the Company.
They still carried out their professional dancing responsibilities;
but new arrangements were made for their education and training.
Theory classes were fixed for the morning and afternoon sessions,
while practical training and rehearsals were fixed for the evening
session.

In April, 1967, the Vice-Chancellor of the University of
Ghana, in order to streamline the operations of the National
Dance Company, the School of Music, Dance and Drama and the
Institute of African Studies, set up a committee to investigate
their academic and professional activities. The one-man member
of this committee was Professor K. A. Busia, a former Ghanaian
Professor of Sociology at Oxford University, England who later
became Prime Minister in the Second Republic. In a letter inviting
him to examine the structure and make recommendations, the
Vice-Chancellor stated the objectives as follows:

> Firstly to clarify the exact aim and objectives and scope of the School
> of Music and Drama, and to determine its place in the framework of
> the University and secondly, to determine which should be proper
> concept of the Institute of African Studies.
>
> (Busia, 1967, p.1)

In his final report which was dated April 7, 1967, Professor

K. A. Busia recommended the retention of the School of Music and Drama, and indicated that:

> Music and Drama transcend the boundaries of Africa, and the inclusion in the Institute of African Studies has limited their scope and orientation. As soon as possible, therefore, there should be established a separate School of Music, Drama and Dance, separate from the Institute of African Studies.
>
> (Busia, 1967, p.4)

While the report made recommendation for the separation of the School of Music, Dance and Drama from the Institute of African Studies in order for the former to have a free hand to develop its academic and training programmes, it suggested that the Company should:

> Remain part of the Institute of African Studies to assist research as a demonstration group, and this, rather than entertainment, should be its primary function.
>
> (Busia, 1967, p.4)

The implementation of the recommendation of the Busia report brought about the separation of the Dance Section of the School of Music and Drama from the National Dance Company. New members were, therefore, recruited to the Company to enable it to serve the research interests in dance of the Institute of African Studies. However, Research Fellows of the Company and the Institute continued to teach dance students for their final examination for the Diploma in Dance which comprised the courses presented in Table 3.

In this examination which took place for the first time at the University of Ghana in June, 1968, two students, Emmanual Ampofo Duodu and William Ofotsu Adinku,[4] emerged successfully and were subsequently employed as Principal Research Assistants Grade II in African Dance in October, 1968. As part of the training and education programmes of the pioneering performers and students of the National Dance Company and the Dance Section of the School of Music and Drama respectively, they were exposed to movement forms of major Ghanaian tradi-

10

TABLE 3

Courses for the Final Examination for the Diploma in Dance

A.   *Written Papers*

(i) Movement Analysis I (Labanotation).
(ii) Movement Analysis II (African Dance Forms).
(iii) Dance History and Criticism.
(iv) Choreography (Principles of Choreography).
(v) Dance and Theatre.
(vi) Music.

B.   *Practical*

(i) Dictation and Sight Reading Tests in Labanotation.
(ii) Assignment in Notating African Dances.
(iii) Performance.
(iv) Choreography.

C.   *Research and Writing*

A minor thesis based on original research in African Dance Forms.

Source: University of Ghana, *Regulation and Syllabus,* 1969, p.13.

tional dances. They learnt the dances and performed alongside traditional dancers. They learnt the various uses of movement and found out that different personalities, according to their status and expected roles, used movement differently. For instance, girls undergoing puberty initiation in Dangme use flowing, flexible and rounded moments in their dnaces in fulfilment of general expectations that women's movement characteristics should be flexible, soft and rounded. Men would use strong, rigid and angular movements in hunting and war dances becuase of the demands of occupation and situation depicting their strong and robust nature. A traditional ruler used mostly "upward" move-

11

ments to depict his monarchical status that he was above "ordinary" men. The students also found out, among others, that movement developments in dances were influenced by the experiences of history, culture, environment and occupation, in addition to the people's aesthetic movement perception.

Insights into these movement forms were necessary for the students because it was envisaged at the time that they would be called upon in future to research into traditional dance forms for educational development as well as create and perform for onlookers who cherish movement forms linked to traditional experiences.

Materials for the students' training were drawn from traditional sources and so they became interested in dance as an element of culture. They also had opportunity to look at movements in terms of their uses — contextual relationship, role differentiations, their musical dimensions as well as their relationships to costumes, make-up and properties.

In the training, it was disclosed to the students that these traditional dances possessed a wide range of movement materials and performance techniques and were assessed and appraised by the people with an inherited set of criteria. In addition, the students realized that, in most cases, people danced separately either facing each other or standing side by side. There were a few occasions when traditional performers got together with a touch or contact. In traditional performances, dancers most often faced the drummers or musicians; the dancers sometimes dance in circular formation with the musicians in the centre. The students also found out that because the dance was an avenue for dramatic expression and for communication between performers and onlookers, there was an exchange of ideas and feelings expressed through various uses of movements. Recreational dancing offered the opportunity to an onlooker to contribute equally actively to the success of the performance if he/she was versatile and so wished.

Today, as the writer sits back to contemplate on the various experiences he went through and review some of the elements and meanings of these dances, he is struck by the significance of these movement forms and the power of those minds that brought the dances into existence. The writer realizes that the organization of movements follows a certain structure with meanings intentionally fused into them, that these movements operate within certain accepted cultural norms which are peculiar to the tradition, and that succeeding creative generations, besides introducing minor innovation and ornaments, seek to maintain a style peculiar to the tradition.

The uses of dance in these traditional societies make the writer believe that dance is a force for revealing ideas about a people's life style and a device for maintaining group solidarity besides the creative uses of movement for aesthetic activity. The traditional dances, therefore, have values for the Ghanaian education system.

The importance of African traditional dance as an educational activity has been stated by Hanna (1965) in her essay *African Dance as Education*. Hanna lays stress on the intrinsic qualities of dances and emphasizes that such expression of ideas and feelings help to indicate various roles of individuals and the value systems of the society: that through performance, individuals come to learn about their expected roles as well as the use of dance for the release of tension. Similarly, Nketia (1965a) and Opoku (1964) have discussed the importance of the dance in Ghanaian traditional institutions as mechanisms for revealing information about the culture of the people.

Although the research activity of Nketia has been centred around ethnomusicology in Africa with emphasis placed on music as a study of culture as well as art form, the relationship of music to African dance forms occupies a high place in his undertakings.

Nketia's dance articles deal with ethnological issues such as the interrelations of dance and music, movement and meanings, role differentiations, spatial organization, costume, make-up and their relationships to dance movements; performance etiquette, evaluative terms and standards of judgement.

On the other hand, Opoku's method has a practical orientation. Opoku's contribution is much restricted to the manipulation of creative models of traditional dances and ceremonies for the developments of theatrical dances. He uses the National Dance Company for developing his new dance forms. His blending of traditional movement forms with ideas of modern choreography has brought about a new dance form for use in the proscenium theatre as well as in the academic institutions in Ghana. His treatment of various choreographic units such as dynamics, design, levels, rhythm, volume, height, width and depth, as well as the portrayal of ethnic passions has marked him out as one of the greatest traditional dance innovators of the country.

The significance of Nketia and Opoku for dance development could, therefore, be characterized into three main areas relating to:

1. The place of dance in traditional societies.

2. Traditional models and their applications in new choreographic works.

3. Appreciation: standards of judgement; appraising, taste and awareness of features.

In order for continuity to be maintained between traditional dance ideas and future developments in dance at the University of Ghana, the underlying meanings of traditional dances and structures which have been exemplified in the academic and creative activities of Nketia and Opoku would be exploited. In this light the three characteristics stated above are further developed into three concepts of (1) Dance as Cultural Activity, (2) Dance as Art, (3) Dance as Aesthetic Activity, and used as a basis for discussion in curriculum planning for the new Bachelor of Arts (Hons.) Dance in Society being envisaged by the writer. Chapter 2, therefore, discusses the significance of the three concepts for African dance studies.

NOTES

1. Left the Comapny at different times within a year of its inception.

2. The School of Music and Drama has since October, 1977 been known as the School of Performing Arts, and operates separately from the Institute of African Studies.

3. Became a student for the Certificate in Dance in October, 1965.

4. These gentlemen are now Senior Lecturers in the School of Performing Arts and hold post-graduate degrees from universities in the United States of America and United Kingdom.

Chapter 2

A CONCEPTUAL FRAMEWORK FOR DANCE EDUCATION

In this chapter, the writer suggests three different areas of investigation of African dance activity. These areas, divided into three sections, are Dance as Cultural Activity; Dance as Art and Dance as Aesthetic Activity. Each area would allow separate investigation into different aspects of the use of dance and its significance for education within the University system in Ghana.

Dance as Cultural Activity

The aim of this section is an understanding of the role and meaning of dance within the cultural expression of the people. This understanding enables students to know the uses of movements and dance in the traditional system.

To enable the Ghanaian students to understand the uses of movements in traditional dances so that they would apply their models in new developments, their education in traditional dances is thought appropriate. It is in fulfilment of this aspiration that an examination of dance as cultural activity becomes important in this investigation.

In order to distinguish the uses of traditional dance forms within the cultural context, discussion centres on three different areas, i.e. ritual, social and recreational. The ritual area links dance to the expression of cosmic principles and helps the mediums in attunement; the social area dwells on the place of dance movements in expressing role differentiations as well as traditional norms, while the recreational type is restricted to the entertainment needs of the users.

In the search for meaning and the significance of dance as ritual activity, one notes that the dance has been based in portraying various laws and principles believed to be found within cosmic nature. The mediums and adherents of the various ritual traditions

16

assume that should they successfully portray these cosmic principles in their dances, it would be easy for them to establish contact with cosmic hosts whose characteristics have been thought to relate to these principles. Attunement with the cosmic laws is, therefore, the desire of all ritual dancers who believe that through such attunement they come to live in harmony with the cosmic forces.

Kple worship among a section of the Ga-Dangme, for instance, is centred around the dance *kpledzoo*. There is no organized worship without the performance of the dance because the gods are dancing gods. The mediums of the *kple* mysteries are believed to be representatives on earth of these gods. So when the mediums dance, then it is in fact the gods who first started the dance in the sky (Kilson, 1971, p.82). During the ritual performance, certain movements are used to entice the gods to come down to earth to interact with the mediums. One of these movements has been referred to as *ngwei*. The arms are raised towards the sky, fists clenched giving the impression of grasping something and the arms pull towards the earth. This movement is performed when possession is anticipated (Kilson, 1971, p.83).

Kple mediums, who are mostly women, portray the gods in their various dances when seeking answers to the various problems that have come to them and their community. One of such problems centres on agriculture. Explaining the significance of dance as an agricultural rite, Kilson said:

> The control of gods over cosmic processes is mimed in certain collective dances at the planting rites... On these occasions when the celebrants return to the shrine form the sacred field, they form a circle in a single file outside the shrine and dance counterclockwise to symbolize the shining of the sun and then clockwise to symbolize the falling of rain.
> (Kilson, 1971, p.84)

Dancing as the core in *kple* ritual portrays the relationship of gods and mediums. It is, therefore, the mechanism through which worship is effected.

Studies in other traditional mystical activities such as the *yeʋe* of the Anlo-Ewes, the *akom* of the Akans, the *klama* of the Dangme, and *lakpa* of the Ga people and their various dances

17

would reveal elements and characteristics that are essential in ritual activity. Characteristics such as the roles of ritual experts, – their training, taboos, costumes, paraphernalia, the music they use, make-up, the uses of movements and dance, the place of the gods and their moral significance are important areas for knowledge for the dance student. Also important to the understanding of the ritual dance is the performance etiquette, performance area, spatial organization, time and context of performance would help a great deal.

In the social context, it would be noted that the use of movements as a form of expression follows definite procedures accepted by the people. The *agbekor* (Awuku, 1984) dance of the Anlo-Ewes is performed during the festival occasion of Hogbetsotso at Anloga to commemorate the great trek of the Anlo-Ewes from enemy territories in Notsie, Togo to their present abode in Ghana. Since the dance is linked to this event, it is performed when the occasion arrives.

The *dipo* (Quarcoo, 1974) of the Dangme is a social ceremony restricted to girls in their puberty stage because the norms demand that they must undergo initiation to inculcate in them the values of womanhood and to prepare them physically and emotionally to face their feminine responsibilities with confidence.

The *adowa* dancer in Ashanti performing within social context, expresses various ideas depicting his/her feelings towards neighbours and onlookers. Nketia reports movement activities in a performance when he said:

> In the dancing ring of the Akan, when a dancer points the right hand or both hands skywards, he is saying 'I look to God . . .'
> (Nketia, 1965a, p.21)

Such use of movements in the Akan society expresses the dancer's attitude towards others in the community. To understand the feeling expressed and the movements used, one has to link them with the social and ordinary behaviour of the Akan people in general. During a performance, symbolic movements are selected and used only when the dancer wants to express an emotional state, otherwise he/she limits himself/herself to general

18

movements which carry no exact meanings.

Within the recreational context, the *gahu* dance of the Anlo-Ewe is meant for women to express their charms and bodily beauty. The wearing of expensive cloths and ornaments attempts to depict the meaning of the dance – "money dance". Initially, men only provided the music for women to dance to; but of late men have been dancing alongside the women.

Other recreational dances with different aims are the *sikyi* of the Akans, the *kpatsa* of the Dangme and the *kpanlogo* of the Ga people.

Dance as cultural activity can be best understood both as embodiment of ideas and feelings and as a structural activity. The structural form such as movements, spatial organization and costumes, communicates ideas; and the dance stands as a vehicle of interaction. The dance performance provides an occasion for action, enabling the participants to demonstrate their abilities as dancers by the way they perform movements and the manner in which they express feelings. Meaning is, therefore, important in these performances if one is to understand the intention of the dancers.

Meaning in the dance also becomes apparent by examing the interaction of dancers and their responses to each other's movements and expression. These interactions may be found in duets, group performances or even in solo dancing when the performer relates to onlookers and musicians. In the duet, one dancer would communicate an idea and the partner would respond with different sets of movements. The dramatic interaction through movements is important to bring out the intended meaning and feeling.

Structural arrangements such as spatial organization of movements also contribute to expression and meaning. Dance would either be linear as found in the *agbekor* dances, serpentine forms common in the *bawa* and *sebere* dances of northern Ghana or circular formation as found in the *gahu* and *dipo* dances. Also important are spinning and turning movements such as the *damba* and *takai* dances, or somersaulting which is common in *asofo* dances. In the Akan society, for instance during a funeral ceremony, a dancer in an *adowa* performance would portray his/

19

her disturbed condition by dancing in a zig-zag formation.

The use of costumes, make-up or properties plays a significant role in expression and communication. Costumes and properties enhance or restrict movement performance; they help to bring out the dramatic effects of a situation. A traditional ruler with a heavy attire on his body and with heavy gold ornaments around the wrists, ankles and knees would have difficulty in moving around; but such restriction emphasizes his role as a monarch — a dignified personality. But a ritual medium wearing only a short skirt and holding a small broom or sword, symbolizing her ritual role, would spin, jump, roll on the ground and run around; these are actions the monarch would not attempt. Different movements, costumes, and properties and their attributes express the character and meanings of the dance and the occasion.

It would be evident from the above discussion that characteristics in traditional dances influence the community because such characteristics express particular meanings which the community understands; individuals, therefore, operate within these characteristics.

In the course of study of dance as cultural activity, methods of appreciation within traditional performance must be given prominence. During a performance, an onlooker walks into the dancing ring and wipes the face of a performer with a cloth or handkerchief. Sometimes after wiping the face, the onlooker and the performer dance together and embrance each other. In another aspect, the onlooker raises the right arm with the third and forefinger stretched and the rest clenched to show appreciation. Others would walk into the ring and fix coins on the forehead of good performers; sometimes onlookers clap their hands.

In a social situation, a traditional ruler sitting in state and watching a performance would show admiration towards a performer by sending a staff-bearer to congratulate the performer.

Various statements are also made to express ones appreciation or feeling for a dancer. In the Akan society, one hears phrases as *nasa da fam*, translated freely as *his/her dance lies on the ground*. This phrase means his/her dance is cool, fluent and relaxed. He/she dances in all its purity. Such a compliment refers to a dancer who, in addition to his/her movement skill and technical virtuosity, shows very excellent understanding of the uses of movements and expression at the appropriate time. In the dancing ring, the dancer is absorbed in the performance and the transfer of movement from one to the other is very effective. Again, the performance of the appropriate movement in response to a musical piece is well considered. His/her understanding of movement norms and creative use of movement in the dancing ring to express feelings and ideas is well considered as a mark of good performance and showmanship.

Other compliments such as *nasa ye petrepetre* meaning *his/her dance is not smooth, not fluent but jerky movements* or *osa nhwehwe anim asa* meaning *he/she dances looking all the time at people instead of concentrating on performance quality* are not good compliments. One may refer to a person in this category as a performer who has simply acquired movement skills without much dancing ability. Such a person usually dances, looking at people to attract admiration, knowing very well that he/she is not a good performer but seeking people's attention. Such a person does not know the dance and so he/she is not absorbed in the performance. He/she is not relaxed and may "hold himself/herself as the stalk of plantain" (Nketia, 1965a, p.20). The plantain is a food crop in the banana family; its stalk is very straight and rigid. Any dancer who inadvertently behaves like the plantain stalk is a bad dancer.

The worst insult is given to a dancer when he/she attracts a statement such as *Emmɔne ho* which is literary translated as *he/she does not smell the dance* or *the dance is not with him/her*. A dancer of this nature is a complete novice who should not be given attention. Someone who has not taken the trouble to learn the dance and yet wants to be seen as a dancer.

Other negative statements refer to the absence of performance quality in men and women. A woman's performance in the dancing ring must indicate rounded movements, soft and fluent with subtle footsteps. When her movements become angular and robust like those of men, it is frowned upon and attracts statements such as *ɔsa mmarima asa* meaning *she dances like men*. Conversely, if a man's dancing movements express qualities like those of women such as softness, fluent and rounded negative

21

comments are said to show displeasure such as *ɔsa te se ɔbaa* meaning *he is effeminate in his dance style.* Men, to express qualities in male dancing, must also express angular, staccato movements. This is well admired and it portrays the characteristics of a man different from those of a woman.

The study of dance, therefore, as cultural expression must take into consideration the meaning of the life styles in which the dance operates. Without these factors as aids to movement activity, it would be very difficult to understand the dance as playing significant roles in cultural behaviour. In education, dance as cultural activity would lead the student into the sentiment and aspiration of the ethnic groups of the country. Such a study would enlighten the student on the values and ideas of the various traditions such as religion, politics, history, rites and working situations. The meaning of these traditions have been embodied in dances such as those of *kple, akom, agbekor, kpatsa, dipo,* and *tapolo.* The study of traditional dance reveals the artistic and non-artistic experience, sensations and meanings that lead to the understanding and appreciation of the behaviours and attitudes of the people and their societies.

Dance as Art

Development of New Dance Forms

The Dance Section of the School of Performing Arts encouraged the development of new dance forms which models have roots in the traditional dance systems. New dances developed must draw on the principles and features of traditional dances but each new dance must have a character different from those of the traditions. With this approach, structural models and ideas associated with traditional dances are used as primary material in creative works.

In the development of new forms of dance, one realizes that it is essential to work with materials which form part of the ordinary experiences of the people in order for continuity to be established between developments in emergent dance societies and traditional ones. It is in this light that much stress is put on traditional dance features and experiences which constitute primary material for existing dances.

22

The teaching of basic dance movements which are selected from different areas of Ghanaian and other African societies for creative education of dance students is greatly encouraged, for students coming from different dance background find that they have experiences and models to which they could easily relate. It is this easy grasp of technique, structures and the ability of students to work with familiar traditional models, and recreating them into new dance forms which is important in the creative process. The personal manipulation of these models, which are imbued with the creative character of the individual composer is greatly encouraged in the development of new dance forms. All these developments, although influenced by traditional dance models, acquire a new status thus linking them with the concept of dance as art which is exemplified in the study of choreography. The development of new dance forms based on choreography will have application mostly in the theatre and educational institutions.

The education of the student choreographer is essential to judicious dance production fused with ideas and design. In addition, the student choreographer must become an observer of life forms and issues and be sensitive to ideas and feelings around him/her.

In choreography, bringing these qualities together to form a dance, the student needs to make selection and then devise a method for projection. Consequently, the technique of selection and projection would form the basis of instruction in choreography. It is by following a plan of study in order to become skillful in the production of dance that makes the concept of dance as art a significant area in the education process. During such an education, the student is guided in the transmutation of choreographic elements into dance work.

The realization that creativity is an innate ability which the student would develop to its fullest capacity is important in the education process. Through such a study, the student comes to recognize various shapes, forms and structures and organizes them into a series of movements to create a dance. Through a systematic study in creativity, the student is guided to express his/her own stylistic way of assembling movement with meanings. This

23

synthesis of ideas and movements leads to sound development of a dance.

The study of choreography implies teaching various traditional and modern techniques to students to enable them to recognize forms and features around them as well as being guided to develop different movement shapes to express meanings. It is such willingness to learn to recognize these creative forms and the desire to transmute them into dances which become an important aspect of the study of choreography. A course in choregraphy would, therefore, help the student to realize his/her objective as a creative personality.

Opoku's Approach to New Dance Forms

The need to produce new dance work out of existing primary materials from traditional dances and ceremonies has been the concern of Opoku since the establishment of the Dance Section and the National Dance Company. His approach has been to create new dances as models of excellence which Ghanaians and other African choreographers will emulate. Below, the writer examines one of these dances by this Ghanaian choreographer and dance educator.

In the repertoire, the "Lamentation for Freedom Fighters" or *Husago-Achia-Husago*, featured prominently. In developing this dance, Opoku made use of traditional ideas and movements. The traditional *Husago* is a ritual dance for deceased members of the *yeve* cult. Opoku borrowed the idea of bereavement from this society.

The following descriptions of the *Husago-Achia-Husago* is divided into three sections namely 1st *Husago* dance, *Achia* dance and 2nd *Husago* dance. They are supported by diagrams to illustrate the dance as observed by the writer.

First Husago Dance

Three men, representing freedom fighters, stand with crossed arms on chest while three women mourners also with crossed arms kneel facing them. Other men and women mourners with crossed arms kneel in a semi-circle facing centre of circle.

24

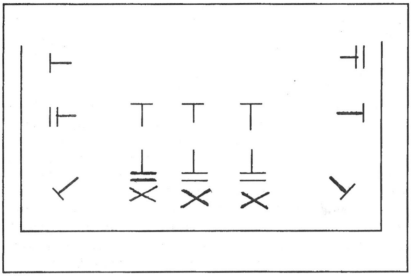

KEY

$\frac{\perp}{\underset{\times}{=}}$ = Freedom fighters standing (Men)

$\frac{\perp}{=}$ = Men kneeling

$\top$ = Women kneeling.

Fig. 1 First *Husago* dance

The three women turn to face down stage and then back to former facing direction, directed by music. In a frenzied mood, they run off stage wailing and beating their mouths with the palm of their right hand.

The three women return to stage dancing with walking steps. The torso is inclined forward high, flexing and contracting, while arms move from first degree forward low flexion to third degree flexion. They move slowly travelling anti-clockwise and arrive in front of the three freedom fighters. Facing stage right, the three women dance forwards and backwards. The rest of the dancers shift their whole body from side to side. Gradually, those kneeling rise and start dancing with emphasis on torso and hand movements. The dance takes them into a circular formation for the *Achia* dance. Fig.1 illustrates the spatial organization of the first *Husago* dance.

Achia Dance

In the *achia* dance, the torso is still bent forward. All the dancers hop forward on the left foot (right foot off the floor) then stamp with right foot in front of the supporting left foot with a clap of hands; both shoulders shrug at the same time. After a number of repetitions of this performance, a new master drum rhythm allows the dancers to hop forward three times on the left foot, and stamp with right foot while both arms thrust forward with a fist alternatively towards the floor. The thrust is done very quickly, first with right arm, then left arm, and right arm again. This last movement series is performed several times. Then the right foot stamps, the left arm is placed on chest and with a clenched right arm in place high position, a turn is performed first anti-clockwise; another stamp and a turn is now performed clockwise. The *Husago* dance begins and slowly they dance off stage. Fig.2 illustrates the spatial organization of the *Achia* dance.

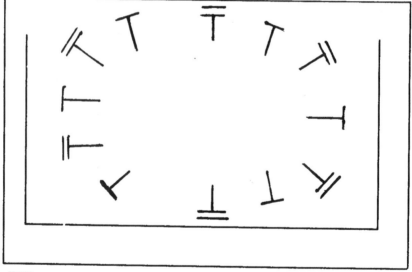

KEY

╤ = Men

T = Women

Fig.2 *Achia* dance

26

Second Husago Dance

The second *Husago* dance now begins and slowly everybody is led off stage by one of the male mourners. The torso is now bent forward, middle knees relaxed. The left hand holding the back of the neck and right arm moves from place middle to side middle continuously. The right leg steps diagonal forward right, then the left leg joins in place; next the left leg steps diagonal forward left, the right leg joins it in place. This movement continues till everybody leaves the stage, and with this the dance ends. Fig.3 illustrates the spatial organization of the second *Husago* dance.

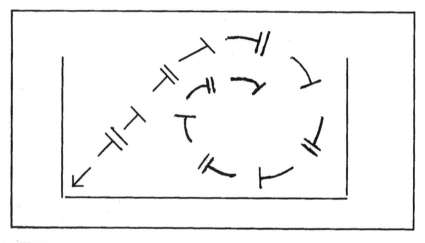

KEY

⊤̄ = Men

T = Women

↙ = Exit

Fig.3 Second *Husago* dance

In general, Opoku's creative work is based upon his research results into the use of movements in various Ghanaian communities. Both conventional and art movements have great influence on him. A gesture such as a clenched hand in place high position has been used in everyday affairs when politicians express power and struggles. In some ritual performance, anti-clockwise and clockwise movements express the idea of the living and the dead (Hanna, 1968, p.24). In *Husago-Achia-Husago,* Opoku combines the idea of clenched hands and circular paths — both clockwise and anti-clockwise — to express the struggles of the deceased fighters as well as those still alive.

Other movements and ideas which have been employed by Opoku dwelt on mourning moods. In real life, a woman will cross both arms on her chest or both hands holding the back of the neck when mourning. When she is completely exhausted from stress and cannot support herself any long she falls on her knees. Sometimes to pay reverence to a high authority, one kneels or squats in front of the incumbent. Opoku employs these movements in his creations. The kneeling of all dancers in front of the three freedom fighters symoblizes this reverence and recognition of their struggles. The crossing of the arms on chest and arms holding the back of the neck in the dance express sorrow and suffering.

All these movement forms have been abstracted from real life behaviour in order to create a new dance. Opoku's work is not dedicated to the traditions but operates in an educational environment and for the theatre.

His work is, therefore, very significant for the discussion of a pure art form because he lays emphasis on manipulation of the feelings and structural forms of dances of the communities into new dance forms. This has become possible because all along he has been operating in an academic institution which functions differently from the traditional environment; but for the sake of continuity of traditional ideas in the academic and theatrical environment, he borrows traditional models.

Opoku's creative work which embodies movement and structural models expressing dynamics, rhythm and spatial designs are abstractions from rituals, ceremonies and practical activities of life. Every element and model is an abstraction. Every emotion is an abstraction from real life experiences. It is what Susanne Langer (1951, p.183) refers to as "aesthetic emotion". This is what Opoku expresses as part of his structural forms.

In looking at Opoku's work carefully, the writer finds traces of influences he has inherited in his knowledge and skill in Choreography and Labanotation. These influences he has carried over the years during his student days at Julliard School of Music, New York and the results of his research into African dance and other dramatic traditions. Such influences has enabled him to operate and work as an authority who has acquired sufficient knowledge and skill. His admiration of Rudolf Von Laban's ideas enables him to incorporate some of Laban's thinking into his works and teachings. Contacts with Martha Graham, Paul Taylor, Merce Cunninghan and other American choreographers have inspired him.

Operating in an institution such as the Dance Section of the School of Performing Arts and the Institute of African Studies enables him to experiment with such knowledge and skill. The outcome has led him to conduct his activities in a professional manner and to relate to fellow artists quite easily and confidently. Artists, therefore, look at Opoku's work for its own sake and examine it for its aesthetic values and nothing else. This is in line with what David Best meant, when he said:

> the artistic is that which is intentionally created or performed for aesthetic value.

> (Best, 1985, p.159)

Best expresses the idea that for an object to be recognized as a work of art, it must be purposefully created with its structures logically linked and expressing the meaning and life issues or forms recognized in the society. For this reason, according to Best, not every structure or phenomenon in real life which observers find to be expressing qualities could become a work of art; rather, it is the qualities which have been consciously synchronized into the work and observed as such.

Opoku's work is an example which fulfils the condition set by Best that a work of art should be intentionally produced to be admired and examined for qualities and meaning.

Dancers who perform Opoku's works also need to acquire the practical skill. It is appropriate that his performers must attain the technical standard for performance. The training of dancers at the Dance Section shapes these dancers in the anticipated skills, developing them into instruments capable of performing complica-

29

ted movement skills. The dancers must perform vividly the structural form and express its intended meaning as envisaged by Opoku. In this way, onlookers come to achieve a sympathetic state with the choreographer, through the performer.

The place of the performer and choreographer is crucial to the new artistic tradition embarked upon in the Dance Section of the School of Performing Arts. For the success of this activity, the first task is the training of performers and creators who would acquire the technique and skill for transforming the elements, structures, and meanings of life around them into new dance forms. With the success of the training programme at the Dance Section, creative personalities have been nurtured to interpret in their work the movement forms and ideas based on African artistic idiom.

Dance, as art in Ghana, is a new development which dates back to the establishment of the Dance Section with its influence from the aims of the National Theatre Movement. The aims encourage creative personalities to help fashion new dance forms for theatrical uses based on traditional African dance values for purposes of continuity. In line with such an idea, the writer accepts that a theory of dance as art is a universal theory, but the interpretation of its meaning in practical terms could only be successful according to influences on choreographers of conventional and art movements of the society in which they live.

It is the feeling of the writer that different societies operating in a theatrical tradition would have different dances embodying the meaning of the concept of dance as art because of differences in creative efforts and cultural differences of the composers. In this same light, Opoku has helped to fashion a new theatrical dance form using movements which he has borrowed from the traditions. His new developments, therefore, fall within the concept.

Dance as Aesthetic Activity

It is important at this stage to indicate the differences in aim between dance as art and dance as aesthetic activity. In examining the domain of dance as art, one lays emphasis on the creative aspect as exemplified in the working approach of Opoku. While Opoku manipulates traditional movements to form his dance, he at the same time embodies ideas and meanings of life forms of the cultures in his work. In examining the dance as aesthetic activity, one emphasizes the structures and subject matter. The analytical approach is, therefore, restricted to the structures, qualities and meanings of the dance movements.

In his contribution to the differences between aesthetic experience and aesthetic activity, Aspin noted:

> We might perhaps find it useful to differentiate the two aspects by saying that one could link the presentation of an object or performance to a spectator. The spectator's perception of it and his response to it as coming under the general heading of "aesthetic experience" whereas his observation, attending, estimation, judging, valuing and so on, we could call "aesthetic activity".

(Aspin, 1974, p.125)

In the quotation above, the word "aesthetic" has been used; but it is important for us to examine the nature of the word in order to apply it successfully in this discussion. The word "aesthetic" was coined by Alexander Baumgarten in the 18th century to denote experiencing, sensory awareness of perception of natural phenomenon (Redfern, 1983, p.12). Perception of natural objects or phenomena thereby enabling the agent to have a pleasureable sensation or the feeling of proportion is believed to be hallmark of the aesthetic.

In addition to the feelings of natural objects, man-made activities such as dance, music, poetry, painting and sculpture were accepted as objects for perception, but with some restrictions. A ritual dance, according to some authorities such as Redfern (1983, p.15), could not be accepted under the concept of the aesthetic because its nature is believed to be functional and operates for the purpose of appeasing a god. It is, therefore, assumed that for a phenomenon or activity to attain the status of the aesthetic, such activity must be produced for the sole purpose of being perceived or contemplated for its own sake.

It is, therefore, important to admit that where an object is

31

to add to aesthetic perception, its form must serve no other purpose and that the aim of the perceiver, in this instance, must be to contemplate and experience the object without any other motive. This reasoning has been the concern of Jorome Stolnitz (1979, p.134) who traced the origin of the development of aesthetic disinterestedness which he argued had helped to bring about appreciation as an autonomous phenomenon.

Aesthetic disinterestedness allows a work of art to be enjoyed in its own ways without any link to the social, political, anthropological or moral situation, because the term "disinterestedness" simply denotes "barely seeing and admiring" (Stolnitz, 1979, p.133). The perceiver must have no other aim or interest beyond the work. The concept of aesthetic disinterestedness does not, therefore, encourage any practical end or aim beyond the object. Neither does it encourage its analysis, criticism or conceptualization. It limits aesthetic interest and disinterestedness to simply pure enjoyment and entertainment without the need to have any understanding or knowledge about the work of art.

In the study of dance as the School of Performing Arts, emphasis is placed on pure enjoyment which falls under aesthetic disinterestedness as well as examing the dance within the concept of aesthetic activity. The examination of the dance as aesthetic activity includes observation, attending, estimation, judging, valuing (Aspin, 1974, p.125). These later aims are different from the aims of aesthetic interest alone which simply denotes "perception alone and terminates upon the object itself" (Stolnitz, 1979, p.134).

With this stand taken to differentiate ideas of aesthetic interest or experience from aesthetic activity, it is essential for readers to note that dance as aesthetic activity would include aims different from dance as an aesthetic experience. Reference to dance as an aethetic activity would, therefore, be examined with the aims of understanding its structures, features or components. It is in analyzing the dance within the concept of aesthetic activity that makes it relevant in this discussion.

In analyzing the dance, one must take into consideration the relationship between the various components which form the structures and qualities expressed in it. These components or

32

observable features express certain qualities which must be recognized. Movement series in the dance may, therefore, be discribed perfectly but if one fails to indicate their character or qualities that these movement series express, one has failed to give a full assessment. For this reason, giving meanings of movements as well as qualities or stating preferences will go a long way towards judgement.

Two influences on appraising dances have been suggested for an orderly judgement: the objectivists' and the relativists' views. Writing on the objectivists' attitude, Suzanne Walther spelt out this position:

> The extreme objectivist critic concentrates on qualitative comparisons of such artistic elements as style, form and technique.
>
> (Walther, 1979, p.67)

The objectivists' position holds that observable features alone are enough criteria for analysis and judgement and that such a position would accommodate no arbitrary criteria from other sources. The objectivists believe such method would standardize judgement; but the relativists also add that:

> Art should be judged according to the value of the culture in which it originates. The relativist position is that beliefs and values are culturally conditioned, they rise within the culture.
>
> (Walther, 1979, p.67)

The relativists state that dance, all over the world, for instance, develops out of the influences of the society's artistic heritage and movements are linked to various ideas and feelings of the society and choreographers make use of these. To judge a dance without any link to the society's feelings and ideas would, therefore, be robbing it of its extended meaning. In this sense, the relativists position holds that the "non-artistic" experiences such as sensations and feelings inherited by the choreographer from his culture fused into his work should be taken into consideration. The fact that dance is an abstraction from experiences and movements of the society means that these influences should be considered when appraising a dance according to the relativists view.

The writer agrees that for a critical analysis of dance in Ghana, one should be guided by both the objectivists and the relativists position in appraising, since dance developments for the theatre and education would be done with movement models, experience and ideas borrowed from various communities as exemplified in the choreographies of Opoku, especially the *Husago-Achia-Husago* previously discussed.

Suzanne Walther has further contributed significantly to the understanding of appreciation and method of dance analysis. Her contribution of the three forms of appraising are significant in helping us to understand the methods of dance analysis. These three forms are:

Description: calling attention to form, and structure in order to ensure that none of the significant detail escapes the observer.

Interpretation: to shed light on meaning, the emotions, style, the symbolic significance communicated in the work.

Evaluation: passing of judgement as to the excellence of the work within a cultural, historical and aesthetic framework.

(Walther, 1979, p.65)

Using the above approach as a guide, the writer now attempts an analysis and appraisal of a critic's report on the National Dance Company's performance of Opoku's works which included the *Husago-Achia-Husago*. This performance took place in Dakar, Senegal in April, 1966.

The full report is stated below:

The National Ensemble of Ghana performed Friday evening at the Liberty Stadium before a large audience. The choreography of the rich repertory entitled "African Dances" carefully designed and accompanied by excellent drumming, was particularly appreciated by the public. The dances representing the folklore of all the regions of Ghana and its neighbouring African countries tell of daily life: domestic and farm labour, war and peace, joy and sorrow. All these scenes, intelligently mimed, won thunderous applause.

Two of the ballets that the audience saw, particularly attracted attention: a War dance and "Husago-Achia-Husago" or Dance Lament.

34

The latter is performed at the funerals of Loved ones. Dancers . . . men and women crouched on the floor with their foreheads touching the ground, undulating their bodies and rocking from side to side while three girls and two boys sang with sadness, to the subtle and unobstructive accompaniment of drums and rattle. Slow at the beginning the rhythm became more broken and percussive while the actors mimed the pain they felt with incomparable agility and virtuousity. But man's life does not consist only of unrelieved grief. It is then that the dancers rose up and looked at life with new hope and serenity.

It is an undeniable fact, and one can say so without any fear of contradiction, that Ghana was one of the best groups since the opening of the world Festival of Negro Arts.

(Martin, 1966)

From the report, the writer makes a selection of the features, exemplify the differences between descriptive, interpretative and evaluative statements as shown in Table 4.

TABLE 4

Analysis and Appraisal of a Critic's Report on the National Dance Company

DESCRIPTION

Dances: men and women crouched on the floor, with their foreheads touching the ground; undulting their bodies and rocking from side to side while three girls and two boys sang; drum and rattles, slow at the beginning; the rhythm became more broken and percussive; actors mimed; dancers arose, drumming.

INTERPRETATION

Designed, appreciated by the public, thunderous applause; sang with sadness; subtle and unobstructive; accompaniment; pain they felt; incomparable agility and virtuousity, unrelieved grief; looked at life with new hope and serenity. Folklore; tell of daily life, domestic and farm labour; war and peace; joy and sorrow; all these scenes; a war dance; dance lament, funeral of loved ones.

EVALUATION

Excellent; intelligently, undeniable fact; fear of contradiction; one of the best groups.

35

The three areas stated in Table 4 above, namely description, interpretation, and evaluation, help to bring out the idea in dance analysis which plays an important role in the understanding of dance as aesthetic activity. Without this appraising process, the concept of dance as aesthetic activity will be eroded. Such understanding includes the functions of observable features that is calling attention to the form, the intended meanings of these features; qualities as well as individual preferences such as how the features and qualities strike the observer. Appreciations or evaluative concept are, therefore, valid area for the curriculum for dance education in Ghana.

The three different areas, namely dance as cultural activity, dance as art, and dance as aesthetic activity, which have been discussed, are essential in introducing the student to knowledge in the dance as associated with the Ghanaian dancing experience — both traditional and theatrical. The Ghanaian and African approach to dance education aims towards the attainment of knowledge in traditional dance activity, as well as proficiency in the creative uses of material and models and critical judgement and appraising.

The approach in dance education is to offer the necessary skills and knowledge which would enable the student to be acquainted with the dances of his society as well as those of others, and be intellectually and artistically prepared for aesthetic and artistic work. To fulfil such aims, one would expect the student to acquire his/her dance education in an organized institution such as the Dance Section of the School of Performing Arts which has had a long tradition of managing educational programme in dance in the country. In such an institution, a student must show three areas of understanding if he/she is to be judged competent and qualified.

The first area deals with understanding of the traditions which gave birth to the traditional dances. These traditions would include areas such as ritual and secular ceremonies and those influencing entertainment. This should be followed up with the mastery of movements of the traditional dances.

The second area would include the use of movements in creative activity. New developments of dances must show evidence

36

of creative uses of models from traditional dances as well as the student's own exploration to show competence in using various elements such as rhythms, dynamics, spatial designs and expression of emotion. Besides performing traditional dances, the student should acquire various performing skills in creative work of other students and faculty members. Individual creative work is intended to deal with varieties of creative and artistic problems. The participation of the student in performing such work would indicate the level of competence reached in practical activity. Besides dance performance, music making is another area of testing a student's understanding of the various instrumental and vocal music of the tradition as well as his/her creative music pieces for the dance.

The third area is understanding the dance, including its historical, ethnological, educational, artistic and aesthetic background. Knowledge gained about the dance should enable students to speak and discuss dance issues convincingly.

Such areas of acquaintance can only be attained in an educational institution where facilities exist for instruction; an institution with competent lecturers who have had many years of experience and knowledge in dance problems and instruction. It is the aim of such an institution to educate and train students to become competent performers, choreographers, music makers and intellectuals. The dance education programme, therefore, becomes an important area in higher education in Ghana.

Chapter 3

A PROPOSAL FOR CURRICULUM PLANNING

Having laid out the ground work for dance study within the three conceptual areas, it is now appropriate for us to examine their various characteristics to help formulate a proposal for course development for a Bachelor of Arts (Hons.) Dance in Society. Courses in this programme would have wholly an African orientation.

The formulation of the proposal is done with the help of three diagrams (Figs. 4, 5 and 6) showing course structures in order to indicate processes for instruction within the three conceptual areas discussed in Chapter 2. These diagrams which characterize the dance experience would suggest methods for practical and theoretical instruction.

Each of the three conceptual areas has a special attribute which is explored in arriving at structural models. Fig.4 lays emphasis on practical and theoretical instruction in African dance within the framework of dance as cultural activity, Fig.5 on the study of choreography as its theme stresses course structures for instruction within the framework of dance as art and Fig.6 on structural models for the study of appreciation within the framework of dance as aesthetic activity.

In formulating a proposal based on dance as cultural activity, we take into consideration, the technique of performance and associated structural models. Within the performance context, uses of movements in different dance styles, and their accompanying musical instruments and songs are considered.

In the traditional societies, movements have been used differently in the dance according to the influence of the people's history, religious beliefs, occupation, social life, as well as the environment. These influences have helped each society to develop its own movement and dance forms. Although it is possible to find similar uses of movement in different ethnic societies, the elaboration of movements in performance would differ from society to society.

Since movements are a common property of the society, their uses as cultural materials in dance forms must follow an accepted norm in order for them to play the role to which they are intended. Individuals who study these movements must acquire the necessary techniques so that their performances would operate within traditional practices. Technical study of movement is, therefore, given a high consideration in the Dance Section of the School of Performing Arts.

Added to technical study of movement is skill development in musical forms. Since music making is an integral part of dance performance in the traditional society, the study of traditional dance would include music performance.

Furthermore, theoretical study of dance is given consideration in understanding African dance. For that matter, the study would lay emphasis on examination of the subject matter of the dance, role differentiation, music, costumes and make-up.

The development of courses for practical and theoretical study within dance as cultural activity is shown in Fig.4 to spell out structural models and processes for instruction.

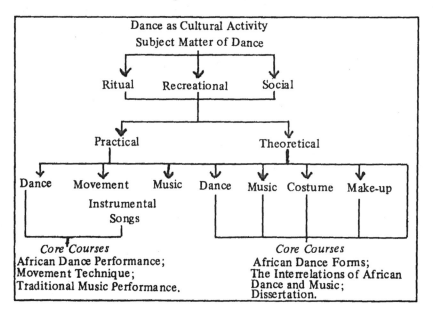

Fig.4 Course Structure for Practical and Theoretical Study of African Dance

From the course structure in Fig.4 the following courses have been developed for practical and theoretical instruction:

African Dance Performance
Movement Technique
Traditional Music Performance
The Interrelations of African Dance and Music
African Dance Forms
Dissertation.

The search for courses continues with structural analysis of Fig.5 within the framework of dance as art. In this area, the study is limited to choreography as a craft. Such a study would enable the student to explore forms of movements to express spatial designs, rhythms and dynamics as well as traditional and modern ideas as subject matter.

In Fig.5 the development of course structure lays out processes for instruction. The choreography course has been developed as a result of the analysis of Fig.5.

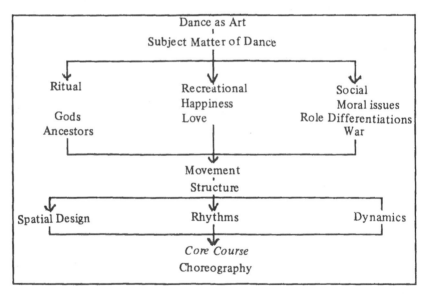

Fig.5 Course Structure for the Study of Choreography

The third area of the dance experience is learning about appreciation within the framework of dance as aesthetic activity.

The study of appreciation requires interpretation of features as discussed in Chapter 2. Appreciation could also indicate the student's preferences such as like or dislike of models but this would be on the basis of description of observable features. In a process of instruction for appreciation, analysis is done within the framework of dance as aesthetic activity shown in Fig.6.

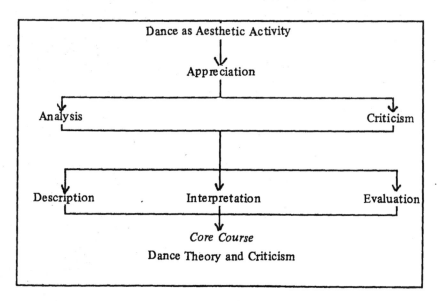

Fig.6 Course Structure for the Study of Appreciation

The structure of Fig.6 leads to the development of a core course: Dance Theory and Criticism. The courses presented in Fig.4, Fig.5 and Fig.6 are outlined in Chapter 4. Added to these courses is documentation which would emphasize Labanotation as a system of writing down dances. A system of documentation is needed to introduce students to the logic of movement scripts for preservation of dances for teaching and learning.

The courses which have been named under the three conceptual areas, i.e. Dance as Cultural Activity, Dance as Art and Dance as Aesthetic Activity, in addition to the fourth course, i.e. Documentation, would form the basis of instruction in the Dance Section; each area would deal with a separate problem and dis-

41

semination of knowledge. Courses associated with these areas would offer the necessary information and skill, which the writer argues, is significant for students at the first degree level.

A proposed outline for the courses developed under the four generic areas is given in Chapter 4. The outline and arrangement of courses into a syllabus show course content, methods of instruction and assessment.

Chapter 4

A MODEL FOR A CURRICULUM IN DANCE EDUCATION IN THE GHANAIAN UNIVERSITY SYSTEM

In Chapter 3, the discussion focussed on the constitutive elements of traditional and theatrical dance. These elements were further expanded into courses which would play a significant role in dance education in the Dance Section of the School of Performing Arts. In the present chapter, the discussion centres on course organization for the proposed three-year programme leading to the award of a Bachelor of Arts (Hons.) Dance in Society.

TABLE 5

Yearly Course Units for a Bachelor of Arts (Hons.) Degree at the University of Ghana

	Course Units		
Department	Year 1	Year 2	Year 3
Major	4	6	6
Minor	2	—	—
Minor	2	—	—

The present course structure for a Bachelor of Arts (Hons.) degree at the University of Ghana covers a three-year period of study. Table 5 shows the arrangement of course units for the three years of study. The first year provides a general study with the student choosing courses from three departments, namely English, Drama and Sociology. A student majoring in Dance would be equivalent to a student majoring in Drama. He/she would, therefore, choose four courses from the Dance Section and two courses each from two minor departments i.e. Sociology and English in the first year of study. The four unit courses from the Dance Section would include two units of theory courses and another

43

two units of practical courses. During the second year of study, the student would choose six course units from the Dance Section, major department, as indicated in Table 6 under Part One Examination. In the third year, the student would select six course units also from the major department as indicated in Table 6 under Part Two Examination.

TABLE 6

Syllabus for the Proposed Bachelor of Arts (Hons.) Dance in Society

Year 1:	First University Examination	Unit
Theory 1:	1. African Dance Forms	1
	2. History of African Dance	1
Practicals:	3. African Dance Performance (Recreational Context)	½
	4. Movement Technique (Recreational Context)	½
	5. Traditional Music Performance (Recreational Context)	1
Year 2:	Part One Examination	
Theory:	1. Dance Theory and Criticism	1
	2. The Interrelations of African Dance and Music	1
	3. Labanotation (Elementary)	1
Practicals	4. African Dance Performance (Social Context)	½
	5. Movement Technique (Social Context)	½
	6. Traditional Music Performance (Social Context)	1
	7. Choreography	1
Year 3:	Part Two Examination	
Theory:	1. African Dance and Related Arts	1
	2. Labanotation (Intermediate)	1
Practicals:	3. African Dance Performance (Ritual Context)	½
	4. Movement Technique (Ritual Context)	½
	5. Traditional Music Performance (Ritual (Conext)	1
	6. Choreography	1
Research Project:	7. Dissertation	1

(Based on *Handbook of Certificate/Diploma Course,*
University of Ghana 1979, pp.63, 70)

The examination for the first year has always been known at the University of Ghana as First University Examination (FUE); the second year examination is known as Part One while the third and final year examination is referred to as Part Two. This arrangement is spelt out in the syllabus structure for the proposed Bachelor of Arts (Hons.) Dance in Society in Table 6 with the value of units shown against each course.

The arrangement of courses for each year within the three-year programme is based on the writer's experiment with course structuring over the years in his capacity as a lecturer in the Dance Section of the School of Performing Arts as well as selecting courses from an existing syllabus which he finds appropriate for the proposed degree programme. In structuring these courses, the writer is guided by the aims of the National Theatre Movement which, in part, suggests that student in any artistic programme including dance should have considerable knowledge and experience in African dance.

The writer suggests, therefore, that the first course should introduce students to the traditional dance forms of the society in order for the students to become acquainted with the meanings of movements, the organization of dance, and the criteria for selecting movements for creating traditional dances. Knowledge gained in this study would enable students to link it with new developments in dance in the emergent society. This study would be done within the course unit *African Dance Forms* and it would go alongside another one unit course *History of African Dance* (Table 6). This course deals with historical influences on dance development.

Practical courses complement the study of *African Dance Forms*. Two of these practical courses are one-half unit courses because they also complement each other. These courses are *African Dance Performance* and *Movement Technique*. The third practical course, *Traditional Music Performance*, is a one unit course. These practical courses lay emphasis on the recreational areas for the first year with studies in such areas as *kpatsa*, *gahu*, *adowa* and *sebere*. The recreational focus for the first year is appropriate because the dances and music are light-hearted in approach. Movement Technique would also concentrate on move-

45

ment associated with recreational performance.

The student, having been introduced to ideas underlying traditional as well as the historical development of dances during the first year of study, now begins to examine various theories of criticism of the dance in the second year for the Part One Examination. Theories about dance as art, dance as cultural activity and dance as aesthetic activity are fully examined. These theories are examined under one unit course, *Dance Theory and Criticism*. Following this course is another one-unit course which aims at explaining the relationships of African dance and music. Since music production plays a significant role in the organization of dance in African societies, emphasis would be placed on this area with the course, *The Interrelations of African Dance and Music.*

Added to the unit courses of Part One indicated in the previous paragraph is *Labanotation* (Elementary). This one-unit course introduces to the student elementary studies in *Labanotation*. This course would prepare him/her for the intermediate level in Part Two.

The three practical courses, i.e. *African Dance Performance, Movement Technique* and *Traditional Music Performance*, continue to be studied but this time the emphasis is placed on dances, movements and musical forms associated with social events. Dances such as *agbekor, fotomfrom, dipo* and *damba/takai* would be learnt in the second year. Musical forms connected with these dances would form part of *Traditional Music Performance*. At this stage, *Movement Technique* would concentrate on movement associated with formal greetings in traditional rulers' courts and other social occasions, as well as different ways of sitting within social events.

Following the practical courses named in the last paragraph is *Choreography*. At this stage, the student begins to learn the rudiments of composition and to develop improvisational skill. The composition of simple solo dances would be started.

In Part Two (year three), a one-unit course, *African Dance and Related Arts* begins with the relationship of dance and other expressive items, e.g. masks, props, costumes and make-up. Study of this course should enable the student to realize the importance

46

of these models and their roles in dance performance.

The continued study of Labanotation (intermediate) for the Part Two Examination is stressed but at this stage the student becomes more involved with the application of elements of Labanotation in documentation of dances.

Included in the courses of Part Two are the practical courses i.e. *African Dance Performance, Movement Technique, Traditional Music Performance* and *Choreography*. Emphasis would be placed on learning dances, musical forms and movements associated with the ritual context. Ritual dances such as *akom, kple/ye ʋe* and their music would form the basis of instruction. *Movement Technique* would deal with cult practices such as greetings, prayers and sitting. The study of choreography now moves into a higher stage, the intermediate stage, with the student composing for duets and group pieces. The choreography would explore the uses of traditional movements and ideas to be supported by creative uses of musical resources by the student.

Finally, for the Part Two Examination, the student undertakes a research project in African dance and related arts and the results are embodied in a dissertation which will be an equivalent to one-unit course.

In structuring this undergraduate programme, the writer intends that as many courses as possible are made available to the student to expose him/her fundamentally to the performing and the scholarly aspects of African dance. Students who aspire to specialize in future will pursue a graduate programme in the chosen area. Such a graduate study is not the objective of this proposal. The aim of this proposal, however, is to further the understanding of traditional dance forms and related arts and the subsequent uses of models in new creative developments. It is, therefore, intended that the development of the undergraduate programme in dance in the Dance Section of the School of Performing Arts would create opportunity for those with career interests shown in the following wing areas in Table 7.

Having stated the aims of the subject, we now describe the curriculum units (*see* Appendix). The arrangement and development of curriculum units above expand the idea that dance education in Ghana should be linked to traditional dance

47

activities. Individual Ghanaians who aspire to become dance teachers, choreographers, performers and researchers within the framework of the National Theatre Movement should seek their dance education at the Dance Section of the School of Performing Arts because it is the only accredited institution in Ghana with a complete academic programme as such.

TABLE 7

Career Prospects for the Holders of the Proposed Bachelor of Arts(Hons.) Dance in Society

Theoretical	Practical	Documentation
	Choreographer	
Instructor		Labanotator
Critic		
Dance Historian	Musician	
African Dance	Performer	
Researcher		

Personnel who would offer instruction in the curriculum would be those with comprehensive understanding of traditional dance forms as well as the aims of the National Theatre Movement. In the teaching programme, the services of non-scholars and scholars would be used.

Non-scholars include the group of persons who have been born into the dance traditions and have acquired expertise in various traditional arts, but do not possess formal educational qualifications. This group comprises musicians, dancers, and movements experts from the various ethnic societies of Ghana. The use of traditional non-literate experts is welcome because the best exponents of traditional artistic forms belong to this group. They have acquired their art unadulterated by foreign ideas and have remained faithful to the aims of the traditions. The Dance Section makes use of these resource persons because of their traditional artistic experience which is difficult to find in the school-educated personnel whose involvement in and understanding of traditional dances and music at the moment is limited.

48

Students, choreographers, performers and scholars would learn from these traditional experts. By this approach, traditional dancing would be linked with classroom instruction thereby allowing traditional models to be successfully employed for new dance forms.

To bring traditional models into classroom learning to enrich instruction, traditional experts would provide the much needed ideas and practical models. These experts would be involved in teaching traditional dances, instrumental music, songs and movement etiquette. By this approach, the students, in addition to learning technique, would be exposed to criteria and standards of judgement of traditional dances, meaning of movement and methods of movement selection for dance developments in traditional societies. Ritual, recreational and social dances would be taught in their traditional ways.

Besides classroom instruction in traditional forms, students would have the opportunity to live in traditional communities for a month or longer where they would be exposed to the natural environment and witness the life styles which influence the development of dances. Students would, therefore, use the occasion to become acquainted with the habits and value systems in terms of which dance is practiced. They would be exposed to other forms of dramatic expression which constitute the embodiments of collective feelings of the communities.

Besides non-scholars, the educational system requires intellectuals who are well versed in the aims of the National Theatre Movement and knowledge associated with traditional dances as well as having expertise in various courses in order to offer meaningful instruction to dance students. Being versed in these areas should be a pre-requisite for accepting academic staff in the Dance Section since the challenge is that whatever new development emerges should be in fulfilment of the tenets of the National Theatre Movement as well as being linked to traditional forms.

49

Chapter 5

CONCLUSIONS

The writer makes a proposal for the development of African dance in education within an African University system using the problems of Ghana. The proposal considers the values of African dance to those who want to employ its models in new creative developments, as well as those who seek an understanding of its forms.

The African dance is accorded recognition by the National Theatre Movement because it reflects the social mores and attitudes of the people; it also expresses their artistic and aesthetic principles. It has played a major role in the life of the people as religious ritual or secular activity. For the African dance to continue to contribute to an understanding of an African way of life, as well as providing resources for new creative developments, the writer makes a proposal for its systematic study at the undergraduate level at the University of Ghana.

The processes for understanding African dance and its related forms have been made within three conceptual frameworks in which instruction and learning would be undertaken. These areas are dance as cultural activity, dance as art and dance as aesthetic activity.

Practical and theoretical study of African dance would be done within the framework of dance as cultural activity. In the practical area, students learn performance technique in different movement expressions within dances. In addition, they learn to perform conventional and ritual movements which express different moods. Added to skill development in movement is training in instrumental and vocal music. The playing of drums, rattles and bells and the singing of selected songs enable the student to learn about musical performance technique.

Furthermore, observation of the dance is important in the learning process. This area examines ideas associated with dance performance. Observation of the African dance, when perfor-

50

mance is in progress, takes into consideration the relationship of music performance and movement expression, the role of participants, the place of costume and make-up, the occasion of performance, as well as spatial designs. The context in which the performance occurs is equally important for the understanding of African dance.

Added to the study of African dance is understanding of historical development of dances. Myths and legends have contributed significantly to the evolution of dance in the African societies. Myths about animals and mythical characters such as the dwarf, the exploits of hunters, as well as migratory events of the people, have contributed to dance developments as well as individual compositions. The study of African dance within context enables the students to relate life styles and cultural issues of the society to the performance of dances. Studying the dance in context also enable the student to examine what the performance means to the indigenous people.

Another area of considerable importance discussed in the proposal is how the results accruing from the study of African dance can be applied in new forms of dances. Such study is done under dance as art. The desire for change in traditional dance forms has been made possible by the introduction of Western education and art forms. Western theatre and ballroom dances have contributed in influencing the new artistic habit of the people. It has enabled them to search for pure theatre. The traditional dances are, therefore, being used to participate in new creative developments for theatrical purposes. In fulfilment of these needs, the student learns methods of choreography as well as the use of traditional resources in new creative developments.

The re-creation of traditional resources has been exemplified in Opoku's works and the proposal lays stress on his working methods as a paradigm and introduces it to the student to show how an African choreographer works. Before creating new dances, Opoku first identifies the characteristics of African dance and, armed with these resources, he begins to create so that there is always a continuity of traditional forms within the context of new dances.

Opoku's experiment is essentially linked to traditional

51

resources because it interpretes and transforms these forms into new creative areas. It actually absorbes traditional forms and in order for these old forms not to become extinct their models are frequently vitalized through re-creation. The student learns how to apply the results of the study of African dance by also examining Opoku's approach in detail.

The third conceptual area for instruction is dance as an aesthetic activity. This area deals with appreciation and it includes analysis and criticism of the dance. The study is intended to contribute to the student's understanding of aesthetic concepts and the language to describe movement processes in a dance performance.

The study of aesthetic terms contributes to the student's ability to offer critical judgement about a performance. The ability to use the appropriate terms for describing feelings and indicating the student's preferences is a mark of sound judgement.

The contribution of dance as aesthetic activity to the learning process cannot be overemphasized. Such a study is a worthy contribution to understanding of description, interpretation and evaluation. It is within this study that the student has access to various concepts in aesthetic appreciation.

The three conceptual areas, i.e. dance as cultural activity, dance as art, and dance as aesthetic activity have provided the framework with which to solve the problem of dance education within the Ghanaian University system. They have provided the formula for a systematic instruction in African dance as well as the resources necessary for creative work. The three conceptual areas have also provided courses for instruction.

The subject, African dance, has explored areas relating to performance and creative techniques, the understanding of aesthetic concepts in addition to understanding traditional dances. All these benefits are made available to the student eager to understand African dance and the application of its resources in new creative work.

The prospect of such a study is that it would also enable the student to understand that dance in African society is the expression of the life of the people because it is an integral part of many religious rituals, social as well as recreational activities. The dance expresses the people's life because it is

Shaped by the values, attitudes and beliefs of the people ... it depends on their feelings, thinking and acting patterns.

(Hanna, 1970, p. 32)

For this reason, the dance contributes to the understanding of meaning of life issues of the society.

Because of its relation to life issues, the study of African dance cannot be done as a solitary exercise in classroom situation alone. For a full understanding of these life issues in which the dance participates, the study would be done when performance is in progress, when performers use the dance as integral aspects of their religious rituals, social and recreational activities. By this field approach, the student comes directly into contact with the dance in its traditional setting and is able to assess the significance of the performance to the occasion and what it means to the participants. This direct field observation would enable the student to witness the live interaction between performers; their acknowledgement both in movement and in text, all of which are important areas for the study of African dance. It is only when performance occurs in context that the student has opportunity to learn performance technique and the manner of showing appreciation by the people.

The study of African dance within context has been emphasized in the proposal to complement classroom instruction. Field observation and participation are stressed because much information on the dances, the relationships of the dance and cultural behaviour, have not been much documented. This is because dance education in Ghana is new and sufficient local experts have not been trained to undertake this exercise. Secondly, a few foreign writers on the dance of Ghana have done so without an elaborate field work and supervision to enable them to understand the cultures that influence the performances. They have written books not with the mind of the African dance performer, but with the mind of the foreign anthropologist, sociologist and notator whose main interest is more towards structural analysis of the performance rather than its subsequent relationship with the

53

contexts. Against this background of lack of objective documentation of the African dance for instruction, the proposal recommends field observation and participation as an approach to objective study.

Since the contexts in which the African dance participates, i.e. the social, religious, historical and anthropolotical, are of great significance to the understanding of the dance, the writer recommends an additional study into cognate areas which would allow the student to have a working knowledge related to these contexts. Studies in related areas such as sociology, religion, history and anthropology are not only desirable but equally important for the African dance student in order for him/her to acquire the necessary technique and tool in which to relate the study of dance. Studies in aspects of sociology may examine dance in terms of social action; studies in anthropology may relate dance to human behaviour; religious studies may link dance to cosmic operations and the moral life while studies in history may look for historical information in dance. (*See* Nketia, 1969; pp. 28–32 for similar suggestions on musicology.) Nevertheless, the significance of these subjects for the understanding of African dance would have to be validated through further research.

The proposal presented for the study of African dance should inspire further research since it is by constantly reviewing the present literature and carrying out further investigation that the descipline of dance will develop.

However, the effective implementation of the proposal in the immediate future may well be delayed by lack of study materials and absence of qualified personnel.

Unlike educational systems in most western countries which rely on a great deal of written documentation of materials for instruction, dance education in Ghana is hampered by the absence of archives with adequate audio-visual items such as films, videos and dance scripts. The development of an archive section in the School of Performing Arts has always been frustrated by lack of funding. Although a small amount of films and videos on dance exist at institutions such as Ghana Broadcasting Corporation, Ghana Film Industry Corporation and National Film and Television Institute, such recordings are mainly extracts of dances.

Another problem is the absence of trained personnel. While it has been the policy of the Dance Section to maintain enough qualified persons to carry out teaching and research successfully, certain areas are still without adequate staffing. The development of areas such as appreciation and labanotation would be greatly handicapped because of problems of recruiting and maintaining staff. It is, however, anticipated that funding would be made available by Government, in future, in order for Ghanaians to embark upon further training and to employ foreign lecturers to meet the immediate problems.

Fortunately, there is no lack of personnel in the traditional dance and related areas because local experts abound. A few past students of the Dance Section, awaiting further training, would be employed to work under the direction of experienced lecturers.

Furthermore, the absence of African dance as an examination subject for the awards of the West African School Certificate and the General Certificate of Education at both Ordinary and Advanced levels would present problems to the Admissions Board of the University of Ghana in determining entry qualifications for the *Bachelor of Arts (Hons.) Dance in Society,* unless other qualifications are regarded as equivalent. At present, regulations for general University entry to first degree programme to secondary school students lays emphasis on the West African School Certificate "O" and "A" Levels or equivalent.

The inclusion of African dance in the curriculum for Secondary Schools towards the examinations identified above would pave the way for serious instruction at higher education level. It would enable pupils to be adequately informed about the dance before their entry to the University of Ghana to pursue undergraduate study.

The problems discussed here would need to be tackled over the years; but the most encouraging prospect is that should the proposal presented in this material be implemented, it would provide the student in the University system with the possibility of systematic study and research in African dance. Such a study should lead the student to become inquisitive and to search for the true value of African dance and its significance for education and theatre in Ghana. All these development would be in fulfilment of the concept of the National Theatre Movement.

Curriculum Units Discussed in Chapter 4

1. Title of Course   —   African Dance Forms.

    Year of Course   —   First Year.

    Duration   —   One academic year of approximately 30 weeks. Class meets twice a week for two hours. Total number of hours a year approximately 120.

    Staffing   —   Instruction would be given by a lecturer of the Dance Section who holds a post-graduate degree in dance including research and teaching experience in African dance and related arts.

                              Complementary instruction would be arranged with resource persons connected with traditional institutions.

    Aims   —   To allow students to examine meanings and principles underlying the development and practice of dance in traditional African societies.

    Objective   —   To gain understanding of traditional dance forms.

    Content   —   Contextual study of dance in African traditional societies; the place of dance in social, ritual, and recreational contexts; meanings and methods of performance — role identities and symbolism in selected dances including the *agbekor, akom, kpatsa* and *damba/takai* (adapted from *Syllabuses and Regulation,* University of Ghana, 1979, p. 63).

    Teaching Method   —   Lecture — discussion. Lecturer leads class in discussing meaning and principles of dances with students contributing to the discussion by previously reading assigned topics. Course would be illustrated with musical recordings, films and video; occasional field trips to traditional areas for observation of traditional dances.

Assessment — One seminar to be presented by each student on assigned topic — Weighting 15 per cent marks. One essay on assigned topic — Weighting 15 per cent marks. One final written examination — weighting 70 per cent marks.

Resources — Access to the libraries of the School of Performing Arts and Institute of African Studies where books and unpublished research materials exist. Visits to major cultural institutes i.e. Ghana Broadcasting Corporation, National Film and Television Institute, Ghana Film Corporation which store audio-visual materials on traditional dances. Short periods of attachment to traditional institutions for study and observation of dances.

Suggested Reading List — Nketia, J. H. 1963. *Drumming in Akan Communities of Ghana.* London: Thomas Nelson and Sons.

Nketia, J. H. 1965. *Ghana: Music, Dance an and Drama,* Accra: Ministry of Information.

Hanna, J. L. 1979. *To Dance is Human: A Theory of Non-Verbal Communication.* Austin: University of Texas Press.

Kwakwa, P. A. 1974. *Dance and Drama of the Gods: A Case Study.* Unpublished M.A. Thesis, University of Ghana, Legon.

Spencer, P. (ed.) 1985. *Society and the Dance.* Cambridge: Cambridge University Press.

57

Williams, D. 1970. The Ewe agbekor. *New Era Magazine*, June, pp. 17–21. Accra: Insight Publications.

2. Title of Course   —   History of African Dance.

Year of Course   —   First Year.

Duration   —   One academic year of approximately 30 weeks. Class meets once a week for two hours. Number of hours for instruction in a year 60.

Staffing   —   Instruction to be given by a lecturer of the Dance Section who holds a post-graduate degree with teaching and research experience in the history and development of dance in Africa.

Aims   —   To develop interest in the study of dance history; that students should understand the reasons underlying the development of dance and its uses to serve the African's quest for artistic and aesthetic satisfaction.

Objective   —   Examination of the chronological development of dance and its underlying theories; application of the knowledge in similar projects.

Content   —   Study of historical events and their influences on the development of dance in selected traditional African societies through oral and written literature e.g. the migration of the Ewe tribe from Togo to the Gold Coast (now Ghana) and its influence on the development of the *agbekor* dances; the Ashanti wars and the developments of the *fotomfrom* and *kete* dances. Concepts, styles and forms of dance in the twentieth century. African theatre through oral literature and written evidences; the National Theatre Movement and the development of the Ghana Dance Ensemble; the development of the High-life dance of West Africa.

Teaching Method	— Lecture — discussion. Lecturer leads class to discuss theories and facts underlying various historical events and their influence on dance developments with students participating by previously reading assigned topics. Illustration with slides, films, and video recordings. Occasional visits to traditional areas and theatres for observation of historical dances.
Assessment	— One seminar to be lead by the student on assigned topic —Weighting 15 per cent marks. One essay on assigned topic — weighting 15 per cent marks. One final written examination weighting 70 per cent marks.
Resource	— Libraries of the School of Performing Arts, the Institute of African Studies and the Balme Library, of the University of Ghana for books and journals. Audio-visual materials exist at National Film and Television Institute, Ghana Film Corporation and Ghana Broadcasting Corporation for viewing and borrowing.
Suggested Reading List	— Adshead, J. and Layson, J. 1983. *Dance History: A Methodology for Study.* London: Dance Book.
	Asare, Y. 1979. *Tapolo-Hunters' Dance of the Nkonya.* Unpublished Diploma in Dance Dissertation, University of Ghana, Legon.
	Hanna, J. L. 1979. *To Dance is Human: A Theory of Non-verbal Communication.* Austin: University of Texas Press.
	Kirstern, L. 1970. *Dance: A Short History of Classical Theatrical Dancing.* Connecticut: Greenwood Publishers.
3. Title of Course	— Dance Theory and Criticism.
Year of Course	— Second Year.

59

Duration	—	One academic year of approximately 30 weeks. Class meets once a week for two hours. Number of teaching hours a year 60.
Staffing	—	Instruction to be given by a lecturer who holds a post-graduate degree in dance with considerable research in dance theory and criticism. Occasional lectures to be given by a lecturer in Philosophy of Art and Aesthetics from the Philosophy Department. Arts critics attached to daily newspapers would be invited to lead seminars.
Aims	—	To develop a constructive critical approach in students towards the evaluation of creative work in the dance. To develop sensitivity to the appreciation of dance as an art form. To develop theoretical thinking in relation to judgement and appraising.
Objective	—	To enable students to become knowledgeable in principles underlying appreciation; to enable them to become dance critics.
Content	—	The relationship of aesthetic features and dance theory to a philosophy of dance as an art form and in education. Evaluative principles and methods of appraising. The place of the dance critics in the society.
Teaching Method	—	Lecture — discussion. Lecturer leads class in discussing theories and ideas of the course with students contributing by previous readings on assigned topics and observation of dances. Use of audiovisual aids such as slides, films and video recordings. Visits to theatres to witness dance performances and discussion with choreographers about their work would be encouraged. Observation of traditional dances.
Assessment	—	One seminar to be presented on assigned topic-weighting 15 per cent marks. One essay on assigned topic — weighting 15 per cent marks. One final written examination — weighting 70 per cent marks.

Resource	— Access to the libraries of the School of Performing Arts and Institute of African Studies for books, journals and unpublished research materials. Recorded dances on video and film exist at the archieves of the National Film and Television Institute and Ghana Broadcasting Corporation. Use of Labanotation texts.
Suggested Reading List	— Aspin, D. M. 1974. Sports and the concept of the aesthetics. In *Readings in the Aesthetics of Sports* (ed. H. T. A. Whiting and D. V. Masterson). London: Lepus Books.
	Adshead, J. (ed.) 1988. *Dance Analysis: Theory and Practice*. London: Dance Books.
	Best, D. 1985. *Feeling and Reason in the Arts.* London: George Allen and Urwin.
	Nketia, J. H. 1965. *Ghana: Music, Dance and Drama.* Accra: Ministry of Information.
	Redfern, B. 1983. *Dance Art and Aesthetic.* London: Dance Books.
	Thompson, R. F. 1973. *African Arts in Motion.* Los Angeles: University of California Press.
4. Title of Course	— The Interrelations of African Dance and Music. (See *Regulation and Syllabus:* University of Ghana, 1979, p.66.)
Year of Course	— Second Year.
Duration	— One academic year of approximately 30 weeks. Class meets once a week for two hours. Number of teaching hours a year 60.
Staffing	— Instruction to be given by a lecturer of the Dance Section who holds a post-graduate degree in Dance with teaching and research experience in traditional dance and related arts. Another lecturer from the Music

61

Department of the School of Performing Arts with considerable research and teaching experience in Music in African Cultures.

Aims — To teach students the relationship of dance and music as traditional and fine art metarials.

Objective — To understand the meaning and structures of dance and music and their relationships in order to apply the results in creative work.

Content — Studies in dance accompaniment and the interpretation of music and sound in bodily movement. Dance and musical communication; the language of drums. songtexts, recital of praise poetry and dirges and their interpretation in dance movements. The function of music in dance; folk or traditional music, popular music or fine arts music, organization of folk music, musical types, performing groups and their music, contextual organization of traditional music: categories of traditional music.

Teaching Method — Lecture – demonstration. Classroom instruction and studio work. Studio demonstration and visits to traditional areas for dance and music observation. Illustration with recordings, films and video.

Assessment — A creative dance piece embodying interpretation of musical structure in bodily movement – weighting 30 per cent marks. One final written examination – weighting 70 per cent marks.

Resources — Books, articles and music recording exist at the libraries of the School of Performing Arts and the Institute of African Studies. Video and Film materials on music and dance would be found in the archives of the National Film and Television Institute and Ghana Broadcasting Corporation.

Suggested Reading List — Awuku, R. S 1984. *Agbekor Dance of Anlo*

Afiadenyigba. Unpblished Diploma in Dance Dissertation, University of Ghana, Legon.

Kinney, S. 1966. A profile of music and movement in the Volta Region, *Research Review* Part 1 No. 1. Legon: Institute of African Studies.

Nketia, J. H. 1965. *The Interrelations of African Music and Dance:* Budapest Studies 1. Musicological Tomus.

Nketia, J. H. 1969. *Ethnomusicology In Ghana.* Accra: Ghana Universities Press.

5. Title of Course	— Labanotation (See *Regulation and Syllabuses,* University of Ghana, 1979, p. 66).
Year of Course	— Second and Third Years.
Duration	— Two academic years of approximately 30 weeks each year. Class meets twice a week for two hours each. Number of teaching hours a year — 120.
Staffing	— To be taught by a lecturer with postgraduate degree in Dance and who in addition possesses at least a teaching Diploma in Labanotation.
Aims	— To give students facility in writing Labanotation; to enable students to acquire the techniques of recording African dances and reading dance scores.
Objectives	— To develop an ability to document dances using the labanotation system; to develop competence in reading scores of notation; to become familiar with methods of documentation.
Content	— Second Year (Elementary): Labanotation symbols, supports, gestures and levels; variation writing in steps and gestures; positions of the feet and jumps; floor patterns.

Third Year (Intermediate): Notation of movement phrases; notation of African Dances e.g. *Kpatsa. adowa, damba;* score writing.

Teaching Methods	—	Lecture — demonstration, plus use of labanotation texts.

Assessment	—	2nd Year (Elementary): Continuous assessment in class work — weighting 15 per cent marks. Examination in sight reading texts in Labanotation — weighting 15 per cent marks. One final Labanotation examination at the elementary level of the Dance Notation Bureau — weighting 70 per cent marks. 3rd Year (Intermediate): Continuous assessment in classwork — weighting 15 per cent marks. Examination in sight reading texts of Ghanaian dances — weighting 15 per cent marks. One final Labanotation examination at the Intermediate level of the Dance Notation Bureau — weighting 70 per cent marks.

Resources	—	Books, journals and Labanotation scripts exist in the Library of the School of Performing Arts.

Suggested Reading List	—	Blum, O. 1973 Dance in Ghana. *Dance Perspective*, 56: 8–55. New York: Dance Perspective Foundation.

Blum, O. 1969. *African Dance and Games.* New York: Selva

Hutchinson, Ann 1977. *Labanotation.* New York: Theatre Arts.

6. Title of Course	—	African Dance and Related Arts (See *Syllabus and Regulations*, University of Ghana, 1979, p. 69).

Year of Course	—	Second Year

Duration	—	One academic year of approximately 30

weeks. Class meets once a week for two hours. Total number of teaching hours a year – 60.

Staffing	–	Lecturer with post-graduate degree in Dance, African Music or Drama in African Societies, with special interest in the relationship of dance and other expressive forms.
Aims.	–	To enable students to understand the relationship of dance and other expressive forms.
Objective	–	To become knowledgeable in the relationship of dance to masks, costumes, props, music and make-up
Content	–	Dance and movement expression; African dance and oral literature; dance and music; dance and masks; dance and props; costume and make-up.
Teaching Method	–	Lecture – demonstration; use of audio-visual materials, i.e. films, music recordings and video. Course would be illustrated with examples of dance performance exphasising the various expressive forms stated above.
Assessment	–	Composing dance embodying the application or oral literature, make-up, costumes, music and masks – weighting 15 per cent marks. One Seminar given by student on assigned topic – weighting 15 per cent marks. One final written examination – weighting 70 per cent marks.
Resources	–	Books, articles, and music recording exist at the libraries of the School of Performing Arts and the Institute of African Studies. Video and Film materials on music and dance would be found in the archives of the National film and Television Institute and the Ghana Broadcasting Corporation.
Suggested Reading List	–	Nketia, J. H. 1965. *Ghana-Music, Dance and Drama.* Accra: Ministry of Information.

65

Nketia, I H 1965. *The Interrelations of African Music and Dance.* Budapest: Studio 1 Musicologia Tomus.

Kwakwa, P. A. 1974. *Dance and Drama of The Gods: A Case Study.* Unpublished M.A. Thesis Legon: University of Ghana.

Kilson, M. 1971. *Kpele Lala — Ga Religious Songs and Symbols.* Cambridge. Massachusetts: Harvard University Press.

7. Title of Course — African Dance Performance.

   Year of Course — First, Second and Third Years.

   Duration — Three academic years. Each year takes approximately 30 weeks. Class meets twice a week for 1½ hours each. Number of teaching hours a year — 90. Total hours for three years — 270.

   Staffing — To be taught by different lecturers and demonstrators of traditional dances. Choreographers occasionally would teach their work.

   Aims — To teach students to acquire the technique of performing different dance styles.

   Objective — To enable students to become proficient in dance performance.

   Content — First Year: Performance styles in three different recreational dances selected from different regions of Ghana, e.g. *kpatsa, adowa. gahu, sebere.*

   Second Year: Performance styles in three different social dance with concentration on dances such as *agbekor, fotomfrom, dipo, damba/takai*

   Third Year: Performance styles in three different ritual dances such as *akom, kple* and *yeve.*

66

Teaching Method	—	Practical training in different dances and choreographic work in dance studio and in traditional areas.
Assessment	—	(Assessed with Movement Technique) Continuous assessment/test assignments in selected dances — weighting 25 per cent marks. Continuous assessment in production participation of two creative works — weighting 25 per cent marks.
Resources	—	Instruction to be done mostly in the dance studio with occasional learning of traditional dances in villages.
8. Title of Course	—	Movement Technique.
Year of Course	—	First, Second and Third Years.
Duration	—	Three academic years. Each year takes approximately 30 weeks. Class meets twice a week for 1½ hours each. Approximate number of hours a year — 90. Total number of hours for three years — 270.
Staffing	—	To be taught by different traditional movement specialists. Course to be supervized by the lecturers of African Dance Performance and African Dance Forms.
Aims	—	To explore various forms of movements in social, recreational, and ritual contexts.
Objective	—	To develop awareness of movements in social, recreational, and ritual contexts
Content	—	Technical study of different ways of greetings, manner of sitting in different societies. Attitude and postures in ritual and social activities, e.g. libation (prayers)
Teaching Method	—	Practical training in the dance studio and in traditional areas.
Assessment	—	(To be assessed with African Dance Perfor-

67

mance). Continuous assessment and test assignments in selected movements connected with social, recreational, and ritual contexts — weighting 50 per cent marks.

Resources — Working mostly in the dance studio and traditional areas.

9. Title of Course — Traditional Music Performance.

Year of Course — First, Second and Third Years

Duration — Three academic years. Each year carries about 30 weeks. Class meets once a week for two hours. Total hours a year — 60. Total number of hours for three years — 180.

Staffing — To be taught by professional traditional instrumentalists and musicians in the employment of the Dance Section. Supervision by lecturers of African Dance Forms, African Dance Performance; the Interrelations of African Dance and Music

Aims — Teaching students various techniques in the performance of instrumental music and traditional songs.

Objective — To become proficient in playing traditional musical instruments and singing songs.

Content — First Year: Playing all the instruments from three recreational ensembles and singing nine songs to accompany African Dance Performance.

Second Year: Playing all the instruments of three music ensembles associated with social events and singing nine songs to accompany African Dance Performance.

Third Year: Playing all the instruments from three ritual ensembles and singing nine songs to accompany African Dance Performance.

68

Teaching Method	— Practical instrumental music and singing at the dance studio. Occasional travels to traditional areas to learn songs and instrumental music.
Assessment	— Continuous assessment each year in techniques of instrumental music performance and singing — weighting 50 per cent marks.
	Test assignments in playing all the instruments of three ensembles plus songs each year — weighting 50 per cent marks.
Resources	— Traditional musical instruments exists at the School of Performing Arts for instruction. Recorded songs on tapes exist in the archives of the Music Department and the Institute of African Studies.
10. Title of Course	— Choreography.
Year of Course	— Second and Third Years.
Duration	— Two academic years of 30 weeks each. Class meets twice a week for two hours. Number of teaching hours a session — 120. Total number of hours for two years — 240.
Staffing	— To be taught by two lecturers one for second year students and another for third year students. Lecturers must hold postgraduate qualification and have considerable experience in choreographic art. Visiting choreographers would hold master classes.
Aims	— To acquaint students with knowledge in compositional elements, such as qualities of motion, directional movements, shapes and dynamics; skill development in choreography.
Objective	— To explore all compositional elements for the creation of dances.
Content	— Second Year: Directional paths and movement shapes; width, height depth and

volume; symmetrical, asymmetrical and oppositional movements to music and sound, improvization of movements to depict various ideas and characters.

Third Year: Making of dances and staging; creative movement development; fusion of movement and music, improvization and its significance for choreography. Creating dances to suit different types of stages.

Teaching Method — Practical instruction and demonstration in the dance studio and on stage.

Assessment — Second Year: Continuous assessment based on approach to study — weighting 50 per cent marks. Test assignment in creating for a solo performance of not more than three minutes — weighting 50 per cent marks.

Third Year: Continuous assessment based on approach to study — weighting 50 per cent marks.

Test assignments in creating dances for duet and a group piece of not more than five and ten minutes respectively — weighting 50 per cent marks.

Resource — Films and video tapes on works of African and foreign choreographers are available at Ghana Broadcasting Corporation for viewing. Film archives of the British Council and the United States Information Services in Accra contain materials on choreographers for viewing.

11. Research Project — Dissertation.

A research project undertaken by the student in his/her final year of study and presented in a written form. The project would report on the organization of dances in ritual, social and recreational events with reference to costume, make-up, music, role

70

differentiations, occasion of performances, areas of performance and movement.

— Weighting on 100 per cent marks.

BIBLIOGRAPHY

Adshead, J. Layson 1983. *Dance History: A Methodology for Study.* London: Dance Books.

Adshead, J. (ed.) 1988. *Dance Analysis: Theory and Practice.* London: Dance Books.

Aspin, D. M. 1979. Sports and the concept of the aesthetics. In *Readings in the Aesthetics of Sports* (ed. H. T. A. Whiting and D. V. Masterson). London: Lepus Books.

Asare, Y. 1979. Topolo – Hunters' Dance of Nkonya. Unpublished Diploma in Dance Dissertation, University of Ghana, Legon.

Awuku, R. S. 1984. *Agbekor Dance of Anlo Afiadenigba.* Unpublished Diploma in Dance Dissertation, University of Ghana, Legon.

Best, D. 1985. *Feeling and Reason in the Arts.* London: George Allen and Unwin.

Blum, O. 1969. *African Dance and Games.* New York: Selva.

Blum, O. 1973. Dance in Ghana. *Dance Perspective* 56: 8–55. New York: Dance Perspective Foundation.

Blum, O. 1973. Dance in Ghana. *Dance Perspective* 56(Winter): 8–55. New York: Dance Perpective Foundation.

Busia, K. A. 1967. *Report on the Re-Organization of the Institute African Studies.* Unpublished report. Legon: University of Ghana.

Hammond, A. 1977. The moving drama of the arts of Ghana. *Sankofa* 1(2 & 3). Tema: Ghana Publishing Corporation.

Hanna, J. L. 1965. African dance as education. In *Impulse.* San Francisco: Impulse Publications.

Hanna, J. L. 1970. Dance and the social sciences: An escalated vision. In *Dance: An Art in Academe* (ed. M. Haberman and T. G. Meise). New York: Columbia University Press.

Hanna, J. L. 1979. *To Dance is Human: A Theory of Non-Verbal Communication.* Austin: University of Texas Press.

Hutchinson, Ann 1977. *Labanotation.* New York: Theatre Arts.

Kilson, M. 1971. *Kpele Lala* – Ga Religious Songs and Symbols.

Cambridge, Massachusetts: Harvard University Press.

Kinney, S. 1966. A profile of music and movement in the Volta Region. *Research Review* Part 1, No.1. Legon: Institute of African Studies.

Kirsten, L. 1970. *Dance: A Short History of Classical Treatical Dancing.* Connecticut: Greenwood Publishers.

Kwakwa, P. A. 1974. *Dance and Drama of the Gods: A Case Study.* Unpublished M.A. Thesis, University of Ghana, Legon.

Langer, S. 1951. *Philosophy in a New Key.* New York: The New American Library.

Martin, L. 1966. *Thunderous Applaase for Ghana's National Ensemble.* Unpublished report. Dakar, Senegal.

Nketia, J. H. 1963. *Drumming in Akan Communities in Ghana.* London: Thomas Nelson and Sons.

Nketia, J. H. 1965a. *Ghana: Music, Dance and Drama.* Accra: Ministry of Information.

Nketia, J. H. 1965b. *The Interrelations of African Music and Dance.* Budapest Studies 1. Musicologica Tomus.

Nketia, J. H. 1969. *Ethnomusicology in Ghana.* Accra: Ghana Universities Press.

Nketia, J. H. 1976. The Role of University in Cultural Development in Africa. (Unpublished). Legon: Institute of African Studies, University of Ghana.

Opoku, A. M. 1964. Thoughts from the School of Music and Drama. *Okyeame* 2(1): 51–60.

Redfern, B. 1983. *Dance Art and Aesthetic.* London: Dance Books.

Spencer, P. (ed.) 1985. *Society and the Dance.* Cambridge: Cambridge University Press.

Stolnitz, J. 1979. On the origins of aesthetic disinterestedness. *Journal of Art and Aesthetic Criticism* XX: 131–143.

Thompson, R. F. 1973. *African Arts in Motion.* Los Angeles: University of California Press.

University of Ghana, 1979. *Handbook of Certificate/Diploma Course.* Legon: University of Ghana.

University of Ghana, 1979. *Regulations and Syllabus.* Legon: University of Ghana.

73

Walther, Suzanne 1979. A cross-cultural approach to dance criticism. In *Dance Research College* (ed. P. A. Rowe and E. Stodelle). New York: CORD.

Williams, D. 1970. The Ewe agbekor. *New Era Magazine,* June, pp. 17–21. Accra: Insight Publications.

INDEX